HERBALIST'S GUIDE TO NATIVE AMERICAN REMEDIES

From Medicinal Plants and Herbs to Ancient and Modern Herbal Remedies for your Effective Home Apothecary Table

Written by SAMANTHA DEERE

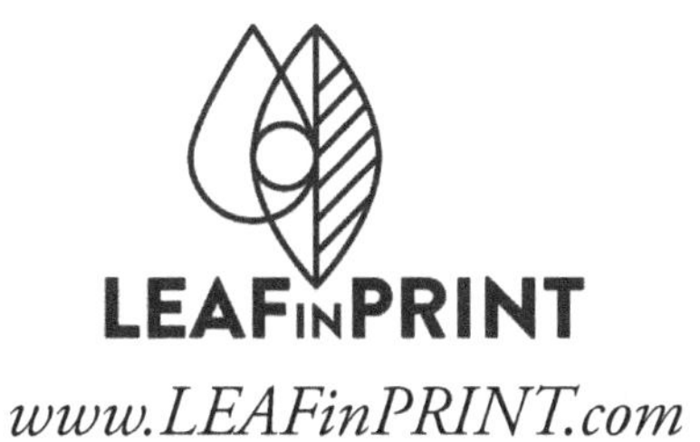

www.LEAFinPRINT.com

Herbalist's Guide to Native American Remedies

ISBN: 978-3-907393-19-2

Contents

List of Medical Herbs and Plants

List of Ailments per Age Group and Ailment

FROM THE SAME AUTHOR

Buy from OUR WEBSITE:

https://www.leafinprint.com/books

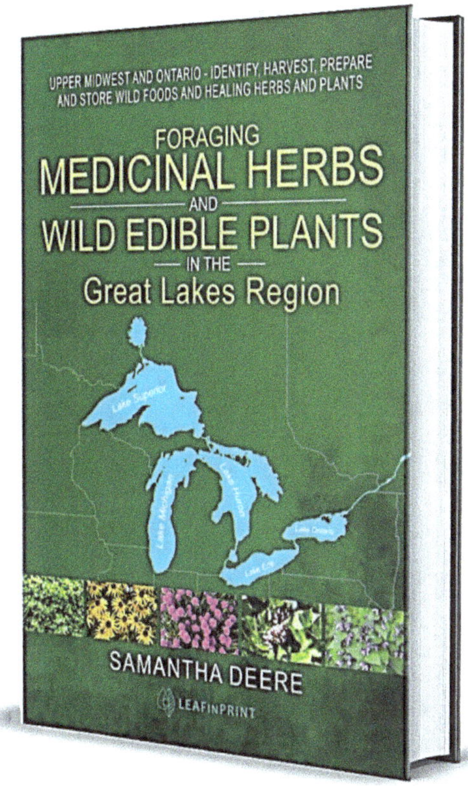

Identify, Harvest,

Prepare and Store

Wild Foods and

Healing Herbs

and Plants

WITH SEASONAL HARVESTING CHART

Foraging Medicinal Herbs and Wild Edible Plants in the Great Lakes Region

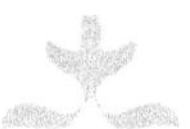

Introduction

Accessing the Native American Ways of Healing

I felt like a walking disaster. Sitting in a coffee shop with a friend, she implored me to see a practitioner. "You need to do something different. You have not found the right doctor to help you," she said. Most of the time, I was an amiable person. However, about a week before my monthly cycle, I became a moody, bloated, unfocused, and exhausted monster that most people wanted to avoid.

The problem seemed to be getting worse month by month. I had started to feel a bit hopeless. Doctors had dismissed the symptoms as 'normal' and told me to take more naps. That was not the answer. At the same time, I knew my life was out of balance. I overworked, ate foods with little nutrition (I often ate meals on the go or while standing), and rarely stopped to enjoy the natural pastoral atmosphere in Vermont, where I lived. How could I put the pieces of my fragmented life back together?

A flyer advertising a local Native American elder gathering stood out to both of us on the coffee shop bulletin board. I had seen the same bulletin before for many years around the same time of year, but I had always dismissed it. Fortunately, at that point, the flyer caught my attention. I needed a new approach, but what would it involve? Could a traditional approach help me? I considered it and decided that the risks were low compared to conventional alternatives. I considered it, took down the number and registered, reluctantly.

Two weeks later, I found myself on a Vermont mountaintop gazing at a teepee with a fire pit in the middle. Packed with seekers like myself, I looked around and saw elders in formal outfits carrying various ob-

jects, feathers, small pouches, and even a small animal's skull. I became nervous. Would they ask me to do something crazy? Then I thought back to my childhood days in a summertime Native American theme day camp. I remembered the prayer we said every day, "Oh great spirit, earth and sky, and sea. You are inside and all around me." The memory soothed me. It would be OK, I told myself, nothing crazy would happen. If it did, I could always walk away.

Participants gathered under a big tent in the Vermont mountains, where twenty Native American elders sat in the middle, forming a circle. They came from various tribes yet had one thing in common; a commitment to restore the value of Native American healing traditions to an audience of around 200 people.

The ceremony began with a prayer accompanied by drum beats that resounded in the ground beneath me. Each drum stroke shook the cool ground covered with fall leaves. A low-pitched soothing chant lulled the audience into an altered state as the sun disappeared. The power of the drums and chants surprised me. I sat and closed my eyes for many, many years for the first time. I just stopped, felt, and listened.

I searched, with expectation, for the grandmotherly figure who would hopefully provide a wise perspective. I could see her in the distance dancing slowly and purposefully with each step.

After the group prayer and following the drum ceremony, the coordinator advised us to proceed to our healer's location. I was the last to arrive and stood in the small circle with people who looked more experienced in attending these sorts of gatherings than I did.

She held a medicine bundle in one hand with feathers and branches that she used to wipe negative energy away from each person in one hand. Very slowly, she went around the circle and stood in front of the participants one at a time. In her other hand, she held a bundle of lit dried sage. After finding a place in the circle, she circled me with sage smoke. A powerful smell filled the area. I watched the smoke drift away and realized how different I felt already. Just the act of slowing down, hearing the drums and the chanting, taking in the cold air, and smell-

HERBALIST'S GUIDE TO NATIVE AMERICAN REMEDIES

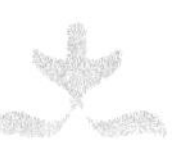

ing the sage smoke brought me into a completely different world. That was only the beginning.

After she smudged everyone and asked us to continue standing. She began to go around the circle. Immediately she stopped in front of me. Slight in stature, she directly addressed me by asking why I was wearing pants. "Pants?" I thought, "What could be wrong with wearing pants on a cold Vermont fall evening? I indicated to her that I felt cold. She just looked at me very calmly. I had not even told her what the problem was. Yet, she already knew.

"Pants," she said, "block the wind from healing the moon cycle." She said that I should wear skirts more often to feel the wind against my skin and learn to walk in the moonlight and pray on the eve of the new moon and the full moon. "If we do not honor the moon, then the moon cycle is disrupted. If you do not honor your moon cycle, it becomes an open wound." An open wound? It sounded so dramatic. Her words shook me. Yet they surprised me because I knew they were so accurate. I was in the grip of the daily grind; honoring anything sacred was the last thing on my mind. However, it didn't feel right, and I knew it. My body knew it, and it was telling me to stop.

She ended on a practical note, telling me that I was deficient in Calcium and needed to eat more greens. That sounded like something my mother would say to me. Smiling to myself, I resolved to give her suggestions a try.

The rituals concluded as the night wore on. I came home and fell into the deepest sleep I could recall having. I woke up, checked the calendar, and saw the new moon cycle approaching. Putting on a skirt and a heavy coat, I went outside, smudged myself with the sage bundle I purchased at the gathering, and said my prayer honoring the moon. It felt a little silly like I was wearing an unfamiliar and cumbersome costume and speaking a foreign language. However, I followed the advice of the elder. Just like breaking in a new pair of shoes, it takes time to make them feel comfortable. So, like a new pair of shoes, I 'tried on' the shaman's suggestions. Increasing my calcium intake, eating greens every day, and stopping to say my prayer to the new moon and full moon worked better than anything I had tried. In two months, I was like a different person. I regained the two weeks of the month I had lost from being out of balance.

Thirty years later, I went through menopause without the symptoms that generally plague women my age. I maintain that the early advice the shaman gave me set the stage for health I continued to enjoy for decades. She became an early model for me as I established my herbal practice. Today, her and modern Native American elders' perspective offer a vanishing yet vital view of embracing traditional healing methods, becoming more resourceful, and leading a balanced and interconnected life.

What this book is about

This book on Native American Herbalist Mastery delivers healing wisdom and herbal approaches to prevent and alleviate common ailments at home. These practices will restore strength, energy, radiance, balance, and confidence. They will help you support yourself and your family as common emergencies arise.

BOOK 1: The Sacred Ways of Native American Healing

- Chapters one through three will lead you through a journey of understanding Native American culture, history, and medical practices.

- Chapter four inspires you to try practical ways to apply these practices to modern life.

Book 2: Native American Herbal Wisdom for Modern Times

- Chapters five, six, and seven guide you through the practical aspects on where to get herbs from and how to store them. Also, it underlines the most important fact that "natural" doesn't necessarily mean "safe" and be good for your health.

- Chapter 8 describes the essential Native American medicine chest that you and your family can efficiently utilize.

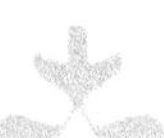

Book 3: How to set up the Apothecary Table that Matches your Needs

- Chapter 9 offers you a toolbox to prepare the herbs so they can be used for the described remedies. This chapter also gives instructions for how much of the common herbs to keep 0n hand, and what to buy additionally when the necessity arises.

- Chapter 10 presents a choice of remedies to cure and prevent common ailments and support wellness for a variety of ages. It instructs you on how to achieve the best results through proper dosage. You will learn how to match the remedy you need by the condition you want to alleviate. If you want to make the remedy yourself, see Chapter 12.

- Chapter 11 gives you an easy reference guide for lists of conditions and herbs to aid them. It features the 'super herbs' or adaptogens that are powerful (substances that heal various types of stress on the body and mind.

- Chapter 12 is your kitchen magician's guide to creating your remedies! You learn about the recipes for the remedies mentioned in previous chapters that total to over forty-five recipes to keep you and your family in the best of health!

Welcome to taking your first steps along the Native American path of healing.

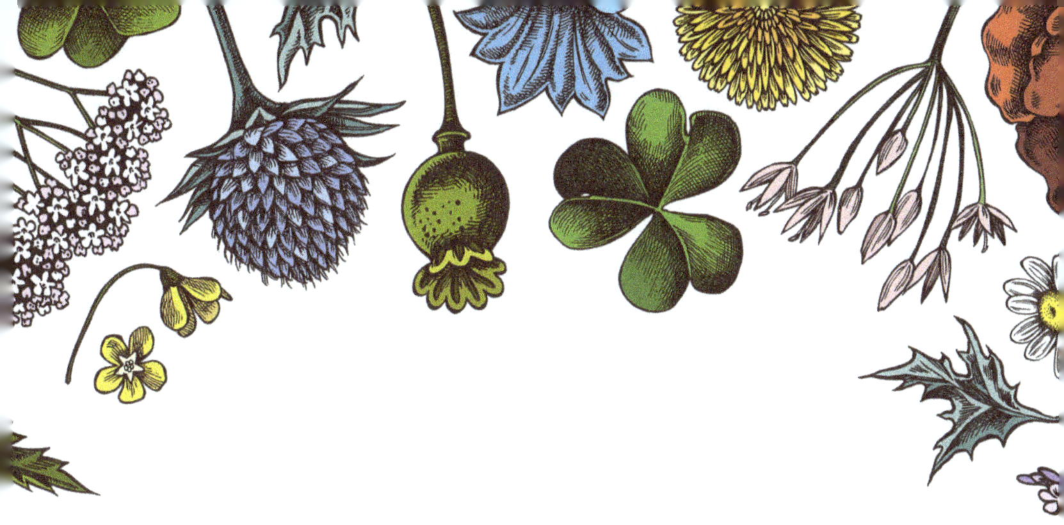

BOOK 1: NATIVE AMERICAN HEALING TRADITIONS

"Humankind has not woven the web of life. We are but one thread within it. Whatever we do to the web, we do to ourselves. All things are bound together. All things connect."

—CHIEF SEATTLE, DUWAMISH

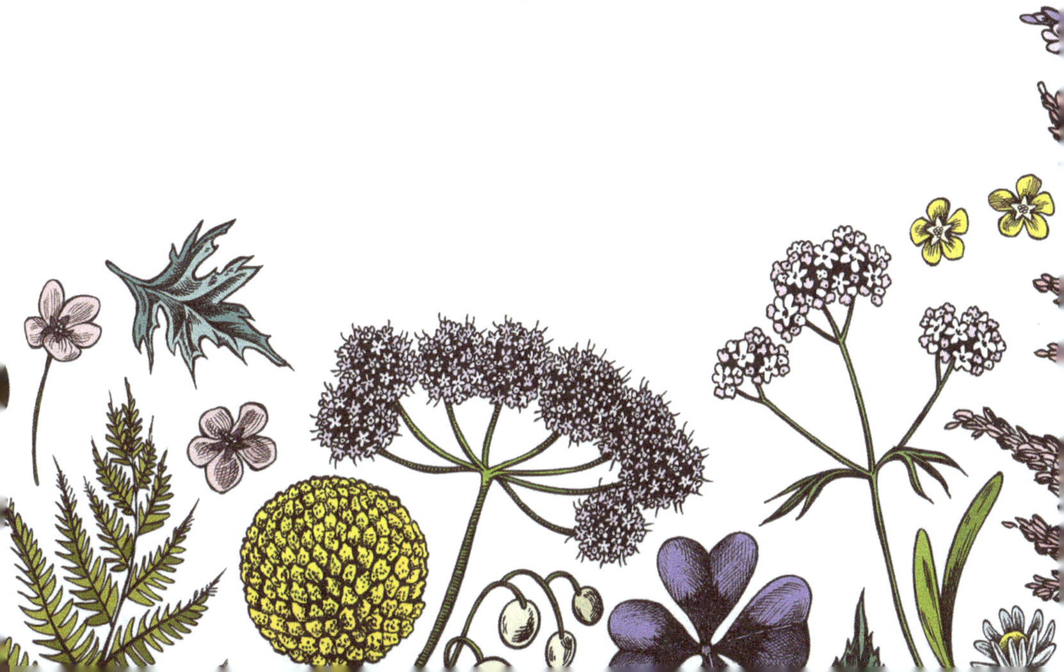

1 History of Herbalism

1.1 The Origins of Herbalism

The history of herbalism begins with the plant itself. Millions of years ago, plants began to populate our oceans. Almost 480 million years ago, plants evolved to cover the earth's topography. Today, there are over half a million plant species. The World Network of Biosphere Reserves has identified 727 biospheres for sustainable development and preservation. It is staggering to think that only one species of modern humans exist within this incredibly complex diversity of plant species. (2)

Traditional healing systems have relied on these plants for thousands of years to restore health and well-being. It is essential to recognize that these conventional healing systems emerged from all continents. Regardless of the geographical location, the premise of each design is the interaction between matter and energy within the person. Specifically, matter means earth, air, water, fire, and ether. All traditional systems believe that humans are composed of these elements and are surrounded by them. These elements must remain balanced within and without for healing to occur.

The relationship between the person and everything around them is fundamental to understanding health, illness, and all of life itself. The state of being of an individual reflects the state of the family and an entire community. The health of a community reflects the web as the whole of life. The Native American herbal tradition, as we shall later see, developed within this comprehensive framework.

As far back as 60,000 BCE, archaeologists have confirmed findings of medicinal vials, uses of culinary herbs, different dyes, cosmetics, and perfumes. These discoveries spread across the globe, from China, Africa, India, Greece, the Americas, and Assyria. During this period, for instance, the tooth plaque of Neanderthals has revealed Yarrow and Chamomile, two prevalent herbs used throughout the world as you read this book.

One can look at the history of herbalism from the texts that have survived the ages, containing precious resources about cultivating, harvesting plants, making remedies, and even case studies showing how natural healers worked with their patients. To a large degree, the history of herbalism and food intersect. We will discover this when reading more about the different Native American tribes and their diet. Humans have used both herbs and spices for their medicinal properties and to flavor food. The spices Turmeric (a root) and Cloves (a seed pod) are good examples of this crossover, and the herb Basil (a leaf) as well.

1.2 Ancient Written Record about Herbalism (500 – 1500 AD)

Surviving texts reveal an astonishing level of complex ancient medical knowledge. The Egyptians created the Ebers Papyrus in 1500, a comprehensive compilation of medical texts containing over 700 herbal formulas. It explains how to use herbs such as Aloe, Garlic, Basil, and Juniper, common substances these days. Similar practices took place in what is now called Indonesia. The Sumatran society in this area produced healing texts on herbalism from 2500 to 700 BC.

The ancient Druid society (Ireland/Scotland) also had remarkable herbal medical knowledge. Multiple discoveries confirm physicians practiced surgeries within stone circles or 'hospitals' for tumor removal. Remains from 1500 BCE confirm using the seeds from the thorn apple for anesthesia. Interestingly Native Americans in certain tribes utilized those same seeds to perform painful procedures. Ironically, the first successful anesthetic in modern times did not arrive until clear ether became synthesized in the 19th century. (5)

In ancient Greece and Rome, Hippocrates, largely considered the father of western medicine and a physician himself, trained other phy-

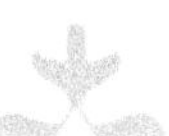

sicians that disease occurred by natural causes rather than curses or superstition. Imprisoned for his far-reaching ideology, he wrote "The Complicated Body" while incarcerated. Healers use the substances and the principles in this book today. Willowbark, for example, a widely used herb for healing fever and pain, is mentioned in his text, as well as Elderberry. This anti-viral and immune-boosting herb became a rare commodity during the global pandemic of 2020.

His guiding philosophy, now known as the Hippocratic Oath, is an extended piece on the integrity of practicing natural medicine. He states, "In purity and according to divine law, I will carry out my life and art" (4). This oath is taken by all types of medical practitioners while in school to this very day. Theophrastus of Eresos 372-286 BC, a pupil of Aristotle, delineated a medical system of plant uses and herbal formulation very carefully. His work remained a standard reference for an impressive 1500 years.

In Ancient RomePliny (AD 77) dedicated seven volumes from his remarkable total of 47 publications to plants and their medicinal uses. He was the first to codify the "Doctrine of Signatures. This doctrine teaches that the color, shape, and even texture represent a part of the human body. For instance, a plant shaped like a lung containing channels similar to it would heal the lung. Likewise, a heart-shaped plant would heal cardiovascular issues.

Traditional Chinese Medicine (TCM) has some of the oldest healing system texts. For instance, the Shennong Ben Cao Jing was recorded in 250 CE attributed to perhaps a collection of individuals rather than just one physician. It reveals a complex system of healing that includes minerals, herbs, barks, roots, animals, fruits, and vegetables. Reishi mushrooms appear in the text and common spices that we use today, such as Ginger, Ginseng, and one of the most famous medicinal foods in the east, mung beans.

Concurrently, as TCM developed, Ayurvedic healing systems, including traditional herbal approaches advanced in the Indian continent Ayurveda means "Science of Life" in Sanskrit. The conventional tribes of Mexico, South America, and Africa had similar systems. Ayurveda dates back to 3300 BCE, at least. There is evidence that ancient east Indians used Turmeric from 4000 BCE.

Ayurveda has four pillars of treatment, yoga, meditation, herbalism, and astrology. It is guided by four primary texts: Yajur Veda, Rig Veda, Sam Veda, and Atharva Veda. Each text teaches the practitioner how to heal the body by balancing the elements that represent the whole of nature. Today, herbs that we consider kitchen herbs like Ginger, Turmeric, Onion, Garlic, and Chile Peppers, figured prominently in Ayurveda and were deemed to be primary treatment herbs. Moreover, as their science advanced, the Ayurvedic herbal compendium included hundreds of herbs and complex formulas.

Physicians, healers, and students traveled between countries, and their knowledge spread. Ayurveda and TCM manifested in other areas such as Egypt, Mesopotamia, the Eastern Mediterranean, and Persia, then over to Armenia, ancient Greece, and finally to old Europe. Cross-cultural exchanges were probably even more common than we assume today.

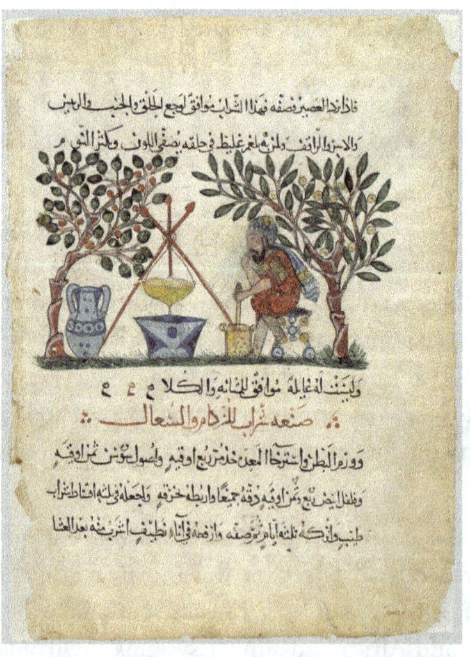

"Physician Preparing an Elixir", Folio from a Materia Medica of Dioscorides dated A.H. 621/ A.D. 1224, 'Abdullah ibn al-Fadl, Figural book painting started in the Islamic world as an art form in the late Abbasid Iraq of the 13th century. (source: *https://www.metmuseum.org/*)

A royal physician named Rhazes in 865-925 resided in Baghdad. He systematized Arabian medicine. Avicenna 980-1037 built upon his predecessor's work and compiled The Canon of Medicine (Kitab al-shi-fa). The Canon brought together all medical knowledge understood in Arab countries. It remained a standard textbook in universities for 700 years until 1650. Meanwhile, in Europe, Abulcasis d. 1013 in Spain, had a notable and advanced using herbal medical practice.

After Rome fell, a six-decade period occurred when scientific exploration, research, and publications ceased. European monasteries primarily protected medical and herbal traditions from 476 AD through 1000 AD during the Dark Ages. Beyond these monasteries, ritualistic herbal practices and tribal magic returned and thrived throughout the globe, as well as the work of some clandestine physicians. As the Dark Ages receded, herbalism again surfaced.

1.3 European Herbalism beyond the Dark Ages — 500 to 1900 AD

Benedictine monasteries during the middle ages continued to protect and carry on the herbal tradition. These monks had enough education to translate Greek and Latin and functioned as physicians. Following the Dark Ages, one monk, John of Gaddesden, produced a substantial text on botanical medicine. During its time, the Medicinae c.1314, also known by its English name Rosa Anglica, broke the silence of the Dark Ages by proclaiming the legitimacy of herbal knowledge once more. His work is a perfect example of cross-cultural influences as it combines herbal, medical, and even personal case studies in Greek, Arab, Jewish and Anglo-Saxon traditions. However, monks were not the only keepers of the craft. Hildegard von Bingen, an extraordinary German nun, seer, and herbalist, wrote Causae et Curae during the 12th century, and people sought her out for cures.

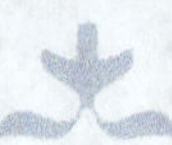

The Grete Herball, first published by Peter Treveris 1526. It is an early modern encyclopedia and the first illustrated herbal produced in English. It is preceded by Richard Banckess unillustrated Herball (1525).

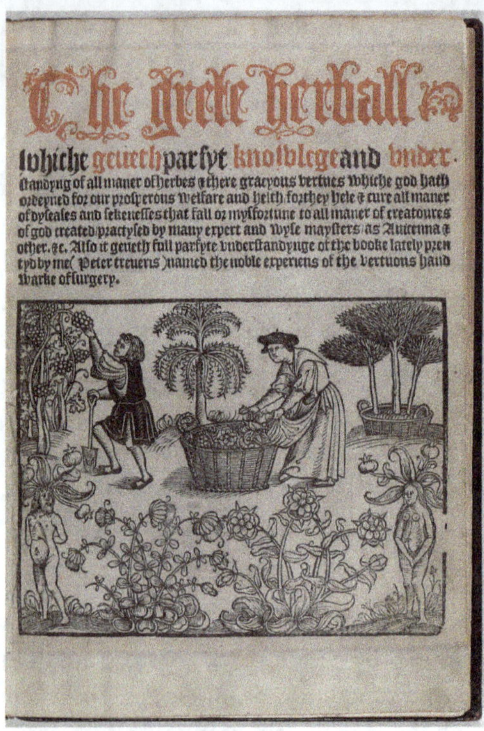

The title page of the 'The Grete Herball' book shows a garden scene, (Peter Treveris 1526). It is an early modern encyclopedia and the first illustrated herbal produced in English (source: *https://www. metmuseum.org/art/ collection/search/365969*).

Following the suppression of the Dark Ages, a revival in herbalism was undoubtedly due. During the 15th to the 18th century, herbalism spread throughout Europe. Scholars translated influential Latin and Greek texts into English. In 1525 Banke's Herbal was published. Many say that it was the first book on herbalism published in English. Soon afterward, in 1526, Grete Herball was printed. For more than 300 years, these seminal works guided generations of practitioners. They taught standard herbal formulations using Rosemary, Lavender, Mint, and Chamomile. You might even have one of these herbs in your possession right now. Botanical science also made great strides during this era. A German physician, Hieronymus Tragus, in 1539, published a comprehensive and exact description of all plants discovered and classified.

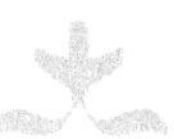

Though the Dark Ages waned from the 1500s to the 1800s, another rather dark trend appeared. Aristocratic classes claimed dominion over herbal medicine and its curative properties. Many practitioners ignored their controls and even practiced in secret. From 1616-1654 Nicolaus Culpepper compiled and produced a substantial contribution to herbal medicine called The Complete Herbal. His work became accessible to all classes and the upper class did not appreciate this. It caused quite a stir during this entire period of herbalism; Culpepper broke the mold by becoming 'the people's herbalist'. The medical community largely disliked him. Yet herbal medical students worldwide study his work.

Although English apothecaries dispensed medicine in the early 1600s, physicians had the exclusive right to diagnose and prescribe. Nonetheless, in 1617 herbalists founded the Worshipful Society of Apothecaries of London. Many of them continued to practice 'illegally,' They also started the Chelsea Physic Garden to preserve a wide range of botanicals. You can still visit this garden today.

1.4 History of Herbalism in the United States and Canada

Around 500 BC, what we know as Native American Indian tribes migrated to North America through Beringia, a land bridge between today's Russia and North America. Their arrival has been documented differently depending on which source you read. For our purposes at this point, we know that they probably brought remedies with them from the east. Native American Medicine has probably been practiced for over 15,000 years. Native ancestry passed down their original tribal and shamanic wisdom generation after generation. Like all healing systems, it was cross-culturally enhanced.

It is ironic that Imperialists influenced the Native populations by introducing certain herbs to them while, at the same time they determined their demise. Likewise it is also ironic that and determined their demise in many respects. It is also ironic that simultaneously native tribes

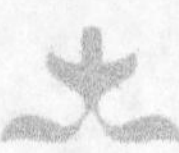

passed on knowledge that kept imperialists, colonists and settlers alive. Master herbalist and teacher Michael Tierra points out that explorers discovered America due to the European demand for herbs and spices. (1)We will continue this story in later sections.

Samuel Thomson (1769-1843) studied Native American Indian medicine in the US and founded Thomsonianism. He combined local herbal practices with the Ayurvedic system and Unani, another word for the Greek system. Soon botanical schools were sprouting up throughout the US. By 1830, Thomsonianism had spread to Europe by Dr. A. I. Coffin. After lecturing and writing about Thompson's system for many years, he combined various herbal philosophies, including Thomsonianism. To ensure the credibility of natural medicine. In 1845 he established the Association of Herbal Medicine. This school evolved into what we currently know as the National Institute of Herbalists in 1864. It is the oldest professional organization of herbal practitioners in the world. However, we must recognize that indigenous populations were still healing themselves in their communities alongside these achievements. Traditional medicine men were probably aware of all the ways their knowledge was being integrated into modern medical schools.

In the US, amongst the enslaved population of African Americans, healing remedies were passed down as a form of survival and medical access for those who had few options. Notably, in the 18th century, some states even made it illegal for the enslaved population to learn about herbal medicine. Harriet Tubman is commonly known for her fearless contribution to the Underground Railroad (hidden channels designed for slaves to escape). However, she was also a well-known herbalist. Likewise, George Washington Carver (1864-1943) was an agricultural scientist and astonishingly productive inventor who studied plants rich in nitrogen, soil rotation, and health. His contributions made it possible for herbalism to survive and thrive at the industrial level.

Herbalism took a distinct turn in the US and Canada in 1904. The Council of Medical Education developed the American Medical Association (AMA). This outgrowth set specific standards for medical schools. If a school could not meet the criteria, the AMA shut it down

   HERBALIST'S GUIDE TO NATIVE AMERICAN REMEDIES

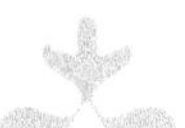

by law. Between 1910 and 1935, more than half of all American natural medical schools, even those affiliated with universities, closed due to the inability to comply with AMA standards. It meant that chiropractic care, naturopathic, osteopathic, homeopathic, and herbal medicine courses were illegal, and these fields could not receive accreditation. Therefore, it is a substantial achievement that herbalism has finally seen a revival over the last fifty years.

1.5   The Revival of Herbalism in Modern Times

The Native American tribal members, like all traditional people throughout the world, used an energetic approach to healing. Their knowledge has survived due to the writings of journalists who lived near the tribes and the oral transmission of elders themselves. Archaeologists have uncovered artifacts, and even the US forestry service has managed to get transcripts of their healing practices. Ethnobotanists have translated their knowledge into materia medica (herbal classifications) to systematize the herbs and reference their procedures to revive these vital substances.

Throughout the wilderness of Northern and Southern Americas remains a storehouse of herbs awaiting discovery. We are fortunate that oral tradition and scholarship preserved the vast traditional legacy of many of these tribes. This preservation allows us to see our healing and connection to the world through the Native American lens when so many long to connect to their inner healer and heal the world around them.

"I see a time of Seven Generations when all the colors of mankind will gather under the Sacred Tree of Life and the whole earth will become one circle again."

—Crazy Horse

We see that era arriving now. Presently, The World Health Organization tells us that almost 80% of the global population depends on herbal medicines for an aspect of their primary care. Germany is quite progressive in this regard; nearly 70% of its physicians prescribe plant-based medication alongside synthetic drugs; plant-based medication is widely available.

Sources

(1)   Tierra, Michael, C.A., N.D., Planetary Herbology, New Mexico: Lotus Press, 1988.

(2)   Hopkin, Alan MA MNIMH, A Brief History of Herbalism, A Brief History of Herbalism — Herbactive Health Clinic, Seen January 14, 2022.

(3)   Yance, Donald R., CN, MH, RH (AHG), Adaptogens in Medical Herbalism, Elite Herbs and Natural Compounds for Mastering Stress, Ageing, and Chronic Disease, 2013.

(4)   National Library of Medicine, trans. Michael North, Greek Medicine — The Hippocratic Oath (nih.gov), 2002.

(5)   Phillips, Graham, "Wisdomkeepers of Stonehenge: The Living Libraries of Megalithic Culture, Vermont: Bear & Company, 2019.

2 History of Native American Medicine

2.1 The Origins of American Herbalism

The first discovery of "America" occurred 15,000 years ago when Native Americans crossed the land bridge and came through Alaska. When European settlers arrived by the 15th century AD, more than 50 million people had already lived in the Americas. Ten million of these people lived in what later was known as the United States.

As these tribes migrated east, they adapted to different areas and climates and adapted to different customs. Today the Native American and Alaskan Native population is around 4.5 million. The US Census Bureau notes that it is about 1.5 percent.

Scholars separate the native population into ten different areas, not including Mexico. The other regions are the Northeast, Southeast, Southwest, California, the vast Plains, the Great Basin region, the Northwest Coast, Arctic, Subarctic, and Plateau. The Native American culture and practices bore many similarities and differences from region to region. Their foods differed, but it is essential to remember that food and food habits were as sacred as ceremony and ritual. They often used the two, food and practice together. The most fundamental thing all tribes held in common was a holy reverence for the natural world and an innate sense of the interconnectedness of all life.

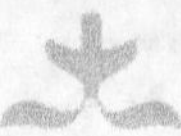

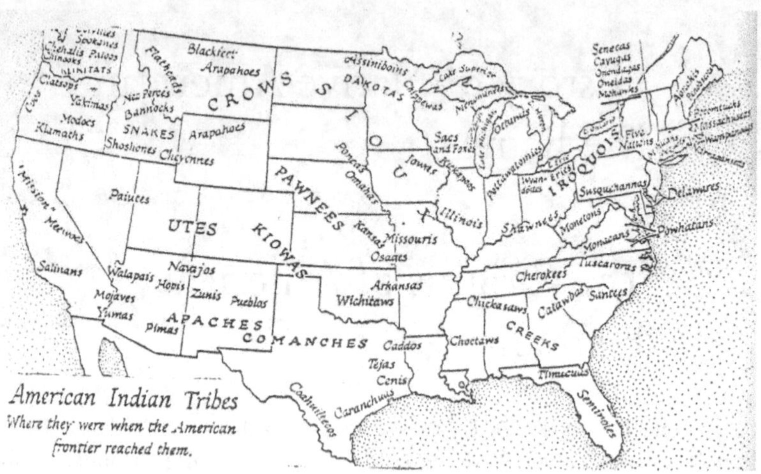

Where American Indian tribes lived around year 1600. Source and more details: *http://genealogytrails.com/main/natives/tribelocations.html*, unknown author and exact date map

2.2 Diversity under Harsh Conditions — Herbalism Arctic Circle Region

Near the Arctic Circle in what we know today as Alaska, Canada, and Greenland, the Inuit and the tribes thrived in a frozen desert — no trees, cold and flat. These nomadic tribes hunted seals and polar bears. The Aleut remained closer to the shore to fish and create small fishing villages along the northeastern shores. Each tribe foraged for wild berries. The unfortunate pattern of oppression and catching diseases from Europeans reduced the population to 2,500 by 1867.

Tribes in the Arctic Circle had inherited their healing traditions orally. The fundamental premise of their medicine was that healing began with the person's spirit, and then this opened the way to understand the disharmony occurring with their environment.

Interestingly the seal and seal oil were a medicine chest in and of themselves. Seal oil alleviated skin rashes, lice, acne, headaches, ear infections, and gastrointestinal disturbances. Berries were fundamental healing companions for gynecological issues and wound healing. Blackberry leaves treated diarrhea, kidney problems, and oral ulcers. Alaskan tribes knew the value of Devil's Club and used it for colds, coughs, and stomach problems. Devil's Club could help mend broken bones and address all issues related to inflammation and congestion. The Tlingit, in particular, believed that Devil's Club had not only solid botanical actions but psychological and spiritual ones as well. Many documented uses of its effectiveness in more severe cases, such as cancer or tuberculosis. (1)

Other common herbs included Willow tree bark, containing acetylsalicylic acid, currently found in many modern painkillers. Alaskan tribes used this bark frequently. They would chew it or boil the bark and make tea. Willow tree leaves made into a poultice could heal skin infections, and healers applied the ash of dried leaves to severe burns and cuts for alleviating skin infections. Native Alaskans used every part of the Dandelion plant. Many other tribes valued Dandelions due to vitamins A, B, C, D. It reaches deeply into the hepatic (liver) ducts to clear liver congestion to alleviate hepatitis and jaundice.

The Subarctic Region required rigor and stamina for survival. The population had to use snowshoes, canoes, and sleds for transportation. Caribou provided their main sustenance, and groups of families followed these herds, settling into portable tents, lean-tos, and then underground dwellings to protect themselves from the harsh cold. When caribou were killed and eaten, tribal members wasted nothing. The killing itself happened in sacred ceremonies, prayers, and blessings.

The main tribes in this region included the Cree, Ojibwa, Naskapi, and Algonquin tribes in the east. The western part became populated by the Tsantine, Gwich'in, and the Deg Xinag. Ultimately these tribes diminished due to fur trading. European traders collected pelts from these tribes, and these exchanges brought deadly diseases along with displacement.

Traditional medicine practiced in these tribes came from deep aboriginal roots, and practices survived through several generations. Healers made pastes or poultices from the plants, juices, infused or decocted teas, and chewed on the raw plants. Their healing process depended on an intimate connection with nature, a solid communal support network, and a central collection of experienced tribal healers. Ethnobotanical literature on the Ojibwa tribe is extensive. A team of prominent ethnobotanists has recorded over 384 plants, including detailed information on medicinal plant applications. (2) Even today, the Ojibwa stand out amongst other tribes as superior healers.

Researchers have gathered that the remaining Subarctic tribes used around 546 different herbs and tree species for healing. They knew the value of herbs we use today, such as Yarrow, a primary fever reducer, and respiratory tonic herb and wound healer. Moreover, they foraged Juniper berries to heal wounds, gastrointestinal and muscular pain, and urinary tract infection. Juniper was a common contraceptive.

The Abenaki populated more stable village habitats. Meanwhile, those who spoke Algonquin like the Shawnee, Fox, Pequot, Wampanoag, Menominee, and Delaware lived along the ocean in fishing villages. They grew vegetables, beans, and corn just a bit further inland. Often both tribes foraged cranberries and stored them during the winter. They made pemmican from cranberries (or other berries) plus fat and dried meat. Hunters and traders carried pemmican on long journeys.

Historically, the Iroquois and Algonquin were not particularly neighborly; their discord fed into further conflict as European colonists arrived and then took sides. Wars essentially scattered the native settlements as tribal members left their lands.

2.3 Sedentary Tribes living on fertile Soils under Mild Climate

The Northeast tribal area had the most prolonged continuous contact with the Europeans. It spanned a large territory from the Canadian border of the Atlantic coast to North Carolina and the Mississippi River. Tribes fell into two categories, the Iroquois language-based population and the Algonquin language-based population. Most of these tribes lived in politically stable villages inland or small shore-based farming communities. The tribes included the Cayuga, Oneida, Erie, Seneca, and Tuscarora, who spoke Iroquois. The Pequot, Fox, Shawnee, Wampanoag, Delaware, and Menominee lived in fishing villages along the seashore and spoke Algonquin. They grew vegetables, beans, and corn.

The Iroquois and Algonquin tribes often conflicted. Moreover, the Iroquois tended to raid neighboring areas. When European colonists arrived, the political situation became more polarized as they took sides during the conflicts. Eventually, the tribes became scattered as western settlers moved towards the west.

Tribal members gathered birch bark to heal joint pain, urinary tract infections, kidney and bladder stones. They taught settlers how to use the May Apple like lemon and boil it for a cathartic (substance for emotional release). Nettles was an excellent remedy for liver and skin ailments. High nutritive tribes would remove the thorns and boil Nettle leaves, eating them like spinach. Another critical staple was groundnuts or Indian Potatoes. Groundnuts were tubers and as crucial as beans, corn, and vegetables. In the 1590s, they were mentioned by Sir Walter Raleigh as he explored the Virginias.

Barberry preparations removed kidney pain and stones and became a sacred object with supernatural powers. Other northern herbs still widely harvested today include Butterfly Weed for viruses and severe respiratory ailments and Goldenrod for all ear, nose, and throat issues. American Elderberry, an antiviral and common Wood Sorrel and Oak bark, root, and leaves, healed severe long-term internal and external infections.

In the Southeast, north of Mexico, five tribes coexisted peacefully, including the Seminole, Cherokee, Creek, Choctaw, and Chickasaw. They successfully raised maize, sunflower, beans, squash, and tobacco. They organized small hamlets where their ceremonies and their daily markets thrived. Over time disease overtook these areas; however, in 1830, the Federal Indian removal act coerced these tribes into relocating. Consequently, the 'Trail of Tears' formed as 100,000 indigenous people made their desperate trek.

Common local curative plants included Sassafras used for blood purification, Jewelweed, an antidote for poison ivy, and insect bites that heals itchy skin within seconds. It contains saponin, a natural anti-inflammatory that we now know functions like cortisone. Frequently, they relied upon Broad Leaf Plantain, one of the most superior dermatological aids available, often called "nature's bandaid. "They chewed or crushed the plantain leaves, applying them to subdermal infections from wasps or hornets. Plantain soothes and repairs the skin while pulling toxins from it. Incredible — most people can find this herb on their front lawn, more towards the driveway because it thrives in rocky areas.

Northwestern coastal tribes, including Athapaskan Haida, Tlingit, Penutian Chinook, Tsimshian, Coast, and the Salishan Coast, Salish had plenty of food, unlike some tribes. They hunted and gathered in the forests and the rivers and oceans. They ate shellfish, whales, otters, and seals. They did not need to travel for sustenance, and so their tribes became very stable within permanent villages containing multiple hundreds of residents. Northwestern tribes operated differently than other tribes through an organized hierarchy that included a powerful chief. Possessions such as blankets, shells, skins, and canoes — and enslaved people — were given to members of certain classes to ensure the tribal class structure.

One of their primary herbs was Echinacea, the incredible lymphatic and blood cleanser. Also, they used Black Cohosh, a favorite herb for supporting both healthy menstruation and menopause. They foraged

American Ginseng for strength and immunity, containing anti-cancer and anti-tumor properties. Saw Palmetto, a plant that could sometimes grow for up to 700 years, alleviated prostate issues. Last but certainly not least, the Northwestern tribes excelled in 'berry medicine'. They used all parts of the blackberry bush for healing. The leaves stopped diarrhea, and the berries alleviated several kidney and gynecological disorders. Berries combined with a green herb like Nettle could help reverse anemia. (7)

2.4 Herbal Traditions of Nomadic Indians on American Plains

In between the Mississippi River and the Rocky Mountains stood a vast prairie region, the Plains. Hunting and farming tribes, mainly Comanche, Blackfeet, and Arapaho, used horses to herd buffalo across the country. They made portable tents from the bison skin taken to different locations. Like the northern tribes who ate caribou, no part of the bison went to waste.

Sadly, white settlers exterminated many of these herds, brought devastating diseases, and taught the Native American to depend on guns, commercial goods, knives, and kettles. Their disrupted culture did not thrive, and most of these tribes had to relocate to government reservations.

Plains tribes favored ceremonies such as recounting dreams and visions, as well as burning sacred plants such as Yarrow and Mullein as medicine. Mullein was a prominent ear, nose, and throat remedy. Mullein also served as natural toilet paper, and the leaves soothed diaper rashes.

Standard practices also included bundling and smudging with plant leaves and stems, like White Sage, Mullein, and Thyme. Smudging was a purification ritual using the smoke from the plant. The practice has Asian origins, and traditional natives likely arrived in this country knowing how to smudge.

One of the most important medicinal foods in the plains region was the prairie turnip used both as a starchy food and poultices to draw out poisons from the skin. (3) Echinacea, though overharvested now, was plentiful during the peak of the Plains Indians' history and is perhaps the most phenomenal lymphatic cleanser and blood purifier available. (10) They used Feverfew, called wild quinine by early settlers, to ease common fevers.

2.5 Arid and Hot Climate — Americas Southwest and California

Native Americans in what we know today as Texas, Utah, Arizona, New Mexico, and parts of Colorado lived two different lifestyles as they formed the Southwest tribal region. The Hopi, Yaqui, Zuni, and Yuma lived in pueblos built from adobe and stone. These complex pueblos had several levels and a central gathering place for ceremonies. The tribes successfully raised squash, beans, corn, and wild onions, pre-serving them for the cold season. On the other hand, nomadic tribes like the Apache and Navajo made temporary homes from mud and bark. Ultimately the Mexican War completely disrupted this area, kill-ing most of the native population. Spanish colonists and missionaries enslaved the rest, forcing them to complete laborious tasks on huge Spanish ranches. In the later 1900s, the remaining people resettled on government reservations.

Southwestern medicinal remedies often included Mint to relieve con-gestion and as an antiseptic. Mints like peppermint and spearmint, often used in teas, can heal headaches and stomachaches because they are versatile herbs. Echinacea, already discussed, was widespread, and Lemon Balm, a primary herb, was cherished as one of the primary sa-cred herbs. Lemon Balm is extraordinary because it subdues ear, nose, and throat issues, reduces infection, and also happens to be an excellent sedative. We will describe it in detail as you work on your dispensary.

To date, many herbalists keep a ready supply of Lemon Balm on hand for children and adults.

It is mind-boggling to consider that California had the largest population before the European conquest. Over 300,000 people lived there. One hundred tribes populated the area speaking more than 100 languages and 200 dialects. Under duress, these migrated during the Spanish conquests. The Hopi, Pomo, Salinas, Shasta, Maidu and Yokuts, and Chumash were the only tribes that influenced this region. California was a peaceful region as triblets existed in the 16th century, organized into bands of hunters/gatherers. In the 1700s, Spanish explorers took trial members into a forced labor mission in San Diego. Slowly this vast population dwindled through disease and assimilation. Although many practices were lost, a revival is currently underway. Perhaps due to the sheer scope of plant species used by the vast tribal population, herbs of the California tribes have not been studied as systematically as other areas of the US.

Native tribes knew that California Evening Primrose, for instance, helps alleviate hot flashes and a host of other menopausal imbalances. Mugwort was an anti-addiction medicine. Yarrow, already mentioned, decreased minor pain like a headache. Sage was a multi-spectrum pain reliever. We understand that Sage has over four dozen different monoterpenoids (chemicals in pants that are antibacterial, antiseptic and antiviral) that are all pain relievers.

California Holly helped cognitive dysfunction (This plant prevailed in Southern California, hence, the name Hollywood). The Valley Oak, full of medicinal treasures, yielded acorns for acorn soup that could rehabilitate anyone in a weak, loose- stooled condition. Oak bark, boiled and made into a poultice, assisted with infections, pulling out sometimes quite deep toxins.

2.6 Great Basin (Rocky Mountains) & Plateau

Great Basin tribes in the Rocky Mountains and the Sierra Nevadas became expert foragers. The Bannock, Ute, and Paiute tribes gathered berries, roots, seeds, nuts and hunted small mammals, snakes, and lizards. They made their homes from willow poles, leaves, and brush, and their settlements were loosely structured and nomadic. Over time white prospectors took gold and silver from these lands, displacing these tribes who frequently had to escape on horseback.

The Ute Tribe has passed down beautiful prayers pertinent to this day to connect to the earth as a healing practice. They were the oldest residents of many Great Basin areas, including Colorado, Utah, Wyoming, Eastern Nevada, and Arizona. Any reader of this book should feel free to use this prayer as a part of their practice if they desire to.

Ute Prayer
From the Uncompahgre Ute Tribe

Earth teach me stillness as the grasses are stilled with light.
Earth teach me suffering as old stones suffer with memory.
Earth teach me humility as blossoms are humble with beginning.
Earth teach me caring as the mother who secures her young.
Earth teach me courage as the tree which stands all alone.
Earth teach me limitations like the ant which crawls on the ground.
Earth teach me freedom as the eagle which soars in the sky.
Earth teach me resignation as the leaves which die in the fall.
Earth teach me regeneration as the seed which rises in the spring.
Earth teach me to forget myself as melted snow forgets its life.
Earth teach me to remember kindness as dry fields weep with rain.

Native American tribes like the Ute often believed that the rainbow had tremendous power and foretold something promising, like a young girl's first menstruation or moon cycle. Walking through a rainbow, for instance, might bring power to a medicine man. The rainbow was inseparable from prayer and symbolized movement between human

and otherworldly spheres. Healers or celebrated heroes could travel between worlds on a rainbow in a ceremony.

Ute tribes harvested the Great Oak, Fiddleneck Ferns, Sage, Barberry (Oregon Grape), Horsetail, and various wild parsley plants. (11)
We will cover these herbs more extensively later. Each one of them
is a perfect addition to the modern apothecary and contains a wealth
of benefits in and of itself. Fiddleneck Ferns appeared in the spring
and were used to alleviate gynecological issues of many types. Horsetail
is a fantastic nourishing herb containing silica, a tissue healer. It also
cleansed the kidneys. Oregon Grape Root is a very reliable broad-spec-
trum antibiotic.

The Plateau cultural area included Idaho, Oregon, Montana, and
Washington. The tribes lived in these areas peacefully along streams
and riverbanks where they would fish for salmon and trout or gather
wild berries, roots, and nuts. Aside from these foods, they gathered cattails from swamps. Young shoots of cattails were consumed in spring,
just like we eat asparagus. Dried cattail roots, when ground, made an
excellent flour. Native Americans in many different tribes combined
the flour with cattail pollen during spring to make pancakes and bread.

Several tribes inhabited the south, including the Klamath, Walla Walla,
Klickitat, Modoc, Nez Perce, and Yakima. Further north, the Skitwish,
Salish, Spokane, and Columbia established permanent dwellings.

Other natives in the 18th century brought horses to the Plateau, which
allowed various tribe members to hunt further from home and even
establish trade routes that crossed the Northwest and the Plains. By
1805 the famous explorers Lewis and Clark came through this territory. Towards the end of the 19th century, the Plateau Tribes relocated
to government reservations as more and more white settlers populated
the region.

Each tribe practiced their medicine slightly differently. Their diets var-
ied as well. However, one strong foundation of Native American tribal
culture was the art of storytelling. Stories even guided medicine men
and healers on using herbs or food in a sacred manner. Accounts, in
general, reinforced the central practice of interconnectedness.

Sources

(1)   Levine, Ketzel (August 11, 2004). "Devil's Club: A Medicine Cabinet for Alaska Tribe". NPR.

(2)   Uprety Y, Asselin H, Dhakal A, Julien N. Traditional use of medicinal plants in the boreal forest of Canada: review and perspectives. J Ethnobiol Ethnomed. 2012 January 30;8:7. DOI: 10.1186/1746-4269-8-7. PMID: 22289509; PMCID: PMC3316145.

(3)   Kindscher, Kelly. "Plant Lore" taken from The Encyclopedia of the Great Plains, University of Kansas, Encyclopedia of the Great Plains | PLANT LORE (unl.edu).

(4)   Tierra, Michael, L.Ac.,O.M.D., "The Way of Herbs," New York: Pocket Books, 1998, pp.131-133.

(5)   Homewytewa, Theodora, "Naturally Occurring Plants Used On The Hopi Indian Reservation for Medicine and Food," National Proceedings: Forest and Conservation Nursery Associations, Utah: USDA Forest Service, 1999-2001.

(6)   Campbell, "Chapter 12. Ute Ethnobotany, University of Montana, chaptertwelve.pdf (umt.edu).

(7)   Kellner, Jessica, "Native Plants and Medicinal Herbs," Mother Earth Living, Native American Plants, and Medicinal Herbs — Mother Earth Living | Healthy Life, Natural Beauty, Seen January 17, 2022.

(8)   History.Com Eds., "Native American History" Native Americans: Tribes and Facts | HISTORY.com — HISTORY, A & E Television Networks, December 4, 2009, updated November 2, 2021.

(9)   Kreiger, Diane, "USC Pharmacist Uncovers Healing Powers of Native Plants," USC Trojan Family, Winter 2014.

(10)   Shaeffer, Elizabeth R. Illus. Grambs Miller, "Dandelion, Poke-weed, and Goosefoot: How the early settlers used plants for food, medicine and home," Massachusetts: Addison Wesley, 1972.

(11)   Lake Thom, Bobby, A Guide to Native American Nature Symbols, Stories and Ceremonies, New York: Penguin Books, 1997.

3   Healing Stories from Native American Tribes

Can you recall a time when you heard a story and felt it settle deep inside, in a transformative way? The Native American population-based their culture on oral tradition and storytelling. They believed that reports could guide and change lives. They played a pivotal role in all phases of life, starting with contemplating creation itself.

Some stories described every situation and every aspect of life. Children heard these stories from infancy and the soothing chants and rhythms during fire-lit gatherings and ceremonies. Stories passed down were like a compass for ethical life, a map for interacting with nature, a navigation device to balance energy with matter. Reports provided strength and courage by introducing heroes and heroines. Storytellers used tales to offer advice in all cases — challenging circumstances, particularly inspiring listeners to go beyond the mundane to the transformative.

Reading some of these stories from different tribes shows how relevant they are to modern life. Some storytellers are current-day elders talking to people starting a healing journey. We have to sit and listen to what these elders and medicine men and women try to teach. The Native American belief system taught that listening brought answers and connection. Is it easy to sit and think of anyone who does not need solutions or connections in today's world? Probably not…

Northwestern
Medicine Comes By Listening

Medicine Man and teacher Bobby Lake Thom describes a modern encounter he had with a friend from the Colville Indian Reservation in Washington State:

"A friend of mine is from the Colville Indian Reservation in Washington State." He came to Spokane to talk to me about some personal problems

one day. He had been unemployed for quite some time, was without money, and was worried about debts. While we sat drinking coffee and talking, I reached into the cabinet and brought out a sweetgrass herb and a Raven wing. I told him a few stories about how hard Raven's life is, but somehow the bird always managed to survive, to 'make it in life. According to our Native myths, the Raven can bring good luck if one is willing to make prayers to the Raven and ask for his help.

So we did a cleansing ritual with the sweet grass, made prayers to the Raven, and threw some food up onto the roof for him. We heard a large squawk a few minutes later and watched a big Raven fly up onto the roof. I told my friend, who was staring in amazement, "See, sometimes it works, huh?" A few days later, this friend called to tell Bobby Thom Lake how he had seen a Raven flying towards his house with food in its mouth. What could this mean? Bobby Lake Thom assured him that it told good fortune was coming. He would receive a gift. Later that day, his friend received an inheritance check in the mail, and on the same day, he got a new job offer. (6)

Plains
Healers Must Respect Natural Laws

Many stories in Native American Traditions teach the importance of having integrity with the natural world. Natural forces and beings bring to power. However, if it is misused, there are always consequences. As a healer, one always has to use energy wisely. Tribal members transmitted these stories to teach their children respect. They also taught that it was critical to have integrity when practicing traditional medicine, obey natural forces and bear the consequences of disobeying natural laws.

The Plains Pawnee tribe told a story of the ceremony of Poor Boy, who marries a chief's daughter. They build a grass hut next to a pond. The girl routinely fetched water and discovered a loon's nest with two small orphaned birds. Although she tries, she cannot capture them. Again, she brings water and overhears the loons, asking why their mother has not returned. She returns a third time, and the loons allow themselves to be caught and taken back to live with the girl and her young spouse.

The orphaned loons speak to the couple, telling them that they will never have children. The couple is quite disturbed and cannot accept their misfortune. However, the loons assure them that the birds will give them powers. However, the story does not end well, for the couple enjoys their capabilities over time yet becomes corrupt. Poor Boy leaves to fight a war with one of the loons as his protector and guide. While he is gone, his wife is unfaithful, and to make matters worse, the wife's lover mistreated the loon that was left behind! Both loons become sick and die from the tragedy, and the couple loses their protection entirely. Poor Boy tries to skin the loons to retain their power by holding on to the skins. It does not work. Poor Boy dies of a broken heart but transmits his knowledge of loon medicine to the chief's son before dying. (1)

Southwest
Medicine Surrounds Us

The following excerpt from a conference held by the US Forestry Service highlights the gifts of a female medicine woman from the Southwest, a wonderful storyteller.

"Good morning. My name is Theodora Homewytewa. I'm from the Hopi tribe…I have no slides, nothing to show you except for what I have here from my heart. That's how I am when I do my work. I am who they call a medicine woman. I collect my plants from the wild. I don't go out and collect an abundance of a certain plant. I go out and see where it is and if what I need is there. Then I pick only what I need… There are different kinds of plant herbs that I use, accompanied by a lot of prayer — always a lot of prayer. The Native American people here know what I am talking about. And when I work on a person, I always know through what prayer she is going to need…a person like myself uses plant life, I gather seeds of a plant that is mature, and other times I get the leaves. Sometimes the root… We go out traditionally at certain times of year…Many of you have lawns out there, and you go and mow them. You just don't care. You just pull those weeds out (Weeds she refers to legitimate herbs for medicinal purposes like Dandelion flowers). To the Anglo people, that's not food. But the Dandelion flowers are really precious to me, so I save them and dry them and give them to a person to calm down. It's got a natural ingredient that calms people

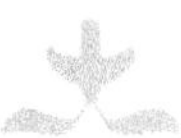

down. So if you are really tired from today go out onto the lawn and find some (laughter). She says how she also boils chaparral root two or three times to make a strong tea. She soaks her clients' feet in the tea to alleviate psoriasis, boils, and abscesses. Whatever you have on your skin, she explains, chaparral is likely to take care of it. (4)

Northeast
One Herb Can Change A Community

The Pine had profound significance for most of the Northern tribes. In the Subarctic Region, the Cree believed that the Pine Root and the Bearded Head were the first two beings on earth. They wield intense spiritual power and pave the way for human birth on the planet. These two powerful beings did not remain forever. They passed on and became stars and plants. (2)

For many centuries Northern tribes made trees from pine needles to prevent colds and coughs. One must remember that these tribes were constantly exposed to the elements, and any simple cold or cough could quickly escalate into something much more severe. This tea had a substantial effect on congestion and respiratory distress. It reduced inflammation due to bronchitis and soothed an irritated throat. Pine needles contain high amounts of vitamin C that support the health of all cells. Vitamin C is a diuretic and enhances immunity, so, understandably, it warded off disease. When the Indians introduced Pine Needle tea to the settlers, the colonists could ward off scurvy, a deadly disease caused by vitamin C deficiency. Pine has an aroma that boosts clarity and concentration and also relieves depression. (1)

Southeast
Traditional Medicine Heals the Whole Person

The 'alikchi practiced Chickasaw traditional medicine. The term signified a medicine man or doctor. The Chickasaw Nation's Heritage and Preservation Division point out that they had a holistic outlook that tied individuals, families, and communities together. Their healing ceremonies and methods were very effective at combining the spiritual, the psychological, and the physical. Medicine men performed chants and sacred prayers over the patient, and the alikchi even provided psychological counseling.

Spirit, mind, relationships to the community, and nature healed during these very intimate times. Every rock, tree, plant, and water contained spirits that tribal members had to be in harmony with to achieve health. Most of their knowledge is gone, yet remaining elders and some journalists have passed down some.

As fate would have it, a doctor in the 18th century Giddeon Linsika lived close to the Chickasaw tribes and recorded their healing methods. He had access to all types of modern medical remedies such as mercury, a popular yet dangerous cure. Still, in the end, his writings show that he found the ways of the traditional Chickasaw healers more effective than his own. A second story reveals the son of missionaries, H.B Cushman, in the 19th century, who recorded conventional healing experiences while living amongst this tribe. He concluded that their medicinal skills were superior to most modern medical doctors, like himself (3)

California
The Power of Native American Medicine Is In Our Backyard

You can walk in your backyard and discover many of the same plants Native Americans utilized all year long. James Adams and his team at the University of Southern California conduct herb walks routinely near campus to teach professional herbalists and the general public that healing is within their grasp.

A dedicated associate professor at the School of Pharmacy, USC in Southern California, Adams tells of his fascinating journey to connect with Chumash tribal herb medicine. His father was a surgeon and Virginia settler who used Native American herbs when medical supplies from England were hard to procure. Adams, a trained pharmacist, remembers being given Sassafras tea for the discomforts of childhood. Later he studied Chumash tribal medicine as a shamanic apprentice for 14 years with a medical woman, Cecilia Garcia. Now internationally renowned, he utilizes his studies to supervise and teach undergraduate students, eager to revive the ancient healing modalities. (11)

In the next section, let's look at ways we can connect more authentically with the sacred ways of Native American life.

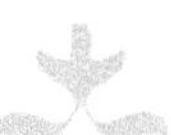

Sources

(1)   Gill, Sam D. and Irene Sullivan, Dictionary of Native American Mythology, New York: Oxford University Press, 1992.

(2)   Drevets, Tricia, The Miracle 'Pine Tree Medicine' That the Native American Indians Drank, https://www.offthegridnews.com/alternative-health/the-miracle-pine-tree-medicine-the native-Americans-drank/

(3)   Chickasaw — TV Video Network, Interview with Dr. Brad R. Lieb of the Chickasaw Nation's Heritage Preservation Division, Winter Fire | Chickasaw. Tv, 2022.

(4)   Homewytewa, Theodora, "Naturally Occurring Plants Used On The Hopi Indian Reservation for Medicine and Food," National Proceedings: Forest and Conservation Nursery Associations, Utah: USDA Forest Service, 1999-2001.

(5)   Anderson, Kat, and Frank K. Lake, Beauty Bounty and Biodiversity: The Story of California Indians' Relationship With Edible Native Geophytes, Fremontia, Vol. 44, No 3. December 2016.

(6)   Lake Thom, Bobby, A Guide to Native American Nature Symbols, Stories and Ceremonies, New York: Penguin Books, 1997.

(7)   Kellogg, Joshua (2010). "Alaskan Wild Berry Resources and Human Health Under the Cloud of Climate Change". Journal of Agricultural and Food Chemistry. 58 (7): 3884–3900. doi:10.1021/jf902693r. PMC 2850959. PMID 20025229.

(8)   Uprety Y, Asselin H, Dhakal A, Julien N. Traditional use of medicinal plants in the boreal forest of Canada: review and perspectives. J Ethnobiol Ethnomed. 2012 January 30;8:7. DOI: 10.1186/1746-4269-8-7. PMID: 22289509; PMCID: PMC3316145.

(9)   Kindscher, Kelly. "Plant Lore" taken from The Encyclopedia of the Great Plains, University of Kansas, Encyclopedia of the Great Plains | PLANT LORE (unl.edu)

(10)   Tierra, Michael, L.Ac.,O.M.D., "The Way of Herbs," New York: Pocket Books, 1998, pp.131-133.

(11)   Kreiger, Diane, "USC Pharmacist Uncovers Healing Powers of Native Plants," USC Trojan Family, Winter 2014

4   Native American Spirituality

The following sections show you how easy it is to call forth the divinity of nature within and without. Long-standing Native American traditions provide you with the knowledge to connect to natural elements. The images chosen reinforce these ideals and the historical context of these practices.

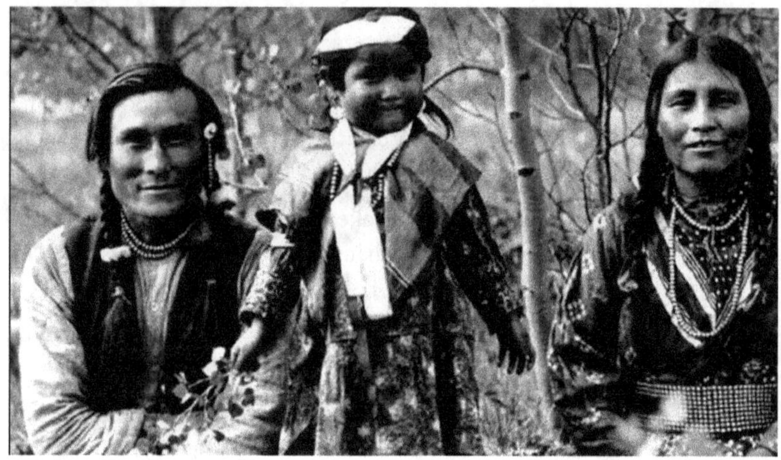

Native American Family (1850-1920s, unknown author)

4.1   The Joy of Reconnecting

We just have to listen. Communication takes place through omens, signs, and mythic religious symbols that create a system of knowledge. To access this knowledge, we do not have to be medicine men or women per se. It is available to an open heart and a willing mind.

Think of it this way — what do we do when a mouse comes into our house or a bird flies into one of the windows in our home? We might be on a walk with a friend. Why does that friend notice a caterpillar is

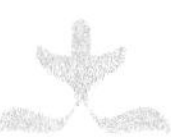

crawling across the ground but not us? When you are driving, is there a hawk circling the field? Why do we see it while the other people in the car remain oblivious?

While we live in a modern world, these signs and symbols interact with us. However, we remain unaware. Nature does not divorce herself from us. We divorce ourselves from her. Maybe we see a moose on the side of the road or an owl flies over our windshield when we are at a stop sign. Suddenly, while getting the mail, a flock of geese comes overhead. There is a sense of awe, but we forget about it and go back inside to open our bills and read our correspondence. Lost in the digital world, we forget the incredible world just across the threshold of our front door.

We have come to see nature as an enemy and try to destroy it. However, this is not the Native American way. On the contrary, traditional Native Americans were immersed in nature and interwove its messages with daily life, work, family, and community. It is ironic that when European settlers came to the Americas, they thought that Native Americans were heathens.

Meanwhile, in diverse languages, in many different forms, Native Americans contemplated creation prayed to the Great Spirit, the Great Invisible One, also called the Great Mystery. They did worship what they thought of, like God and all God created. It makes sense that they prayed to the Sun, Moon, Rivers, Stars, Lakes, Trees, Plants, Birds, Fish, Mammals, Water, and Rocks. For them, it was no different than praying to the universal God.

Native American life was more about listening intensely to all that surrounded them than creating noise and distractions that brought them away from their nature. Listening skills helped them connect, but they also offered protection by encouraging keen observation and foresight.

Native American spirituality was routinely dismissed. Native tribes endured persecution for many centuries. Finally, in 1978, the American Religious Freedom Act became federal law. It protected the rights of tribal members to claim sacred sites objects and worship freely using their traditional ceremonies and rituals. **(8)**

4.2 The Meaning of 'Medicine' for Native Americans

Medicine to the Native Americans was not only a substance. All forms of life held medicinal aspects. Knowing stories, prayers, practicing rituals, and having visions and spirits gave people power. Knowledge produced power, and power became medicine. Herbal substances represented one of many aspects of this power.

Medicine, like any power, could be used for good or to harm. However, sorcery from tribe to tribe was frowned upon as a violation of the sacred way. In general, tribal ways were gentle, peaceful, harmonious and fostered. Tribal members smoked herbs, and medicine men rubbed the ashes from herbs on a person who had ailments. Rocks became medicine when they were heated, the shaman evokes their powers, and the rocks communicated with those participating in the healing ritual.

Most tribes believed that animals could make the medicine in different forms or transform their spirit into medicine. Water was always thought of as powerful medicine, even sweat itself as it was a form of water. For this reason, a sweat lodge ceremony, for instance, heals through its elemental power. The Lakota Sweat is considered medicine. Animals would deliver healing substances—Winabojo is a trickster deity known as a cultural hero who brings medicine to humans. The Cree and Ojibwa believed the Thunder, or 'Pineesi' as they called it, was a powerful form of medicine. Many tribes had a unique name for Thunder to signify respect for its intensity. (2)

This book introduces the most common form of Native American medicine, translated into modern herbal practices. Tribal practices vary widely. Healers gave treatments in a comprehensive sacred context. It was not just a pill or a particular dosage or procedure designed to eliminate a symptom. 'Where did it come from', the Native Americans asked. Only after deeper inquiry, the medicine man or healer administer herbal preparation. In Book 3, we'll focus on herbal medicinal substances and home preparation. However, first, begin to place your

ailments into your own daily context. Native American practices must become accessible in your everyday life.

Medicine Men and Women

How does someone become a medicine man or woman? Mainly it occurs when one receives an inner calling and elders instruct them. Sometimes the process used to last more than a decade. Bobby Lake Thom, born from a Karuk father, Charles "Red Hawk '' Thom, and a mother, Ruby, part Seneca, part Cherokee, and Caucasian, tells his own story.

His father inherited the Red Hawk totem from a medicine man and his grandfather. The sacred call was so strong that he felt it as a child. He dreamt of the hawk. It watched over him, and it protected him. It visited him during sweat lodge ceremonies and provided a chant to sing as a form of personal power. He sang during hunting, ceremonies, and while counseling others. The Red Hawk was used as a line or connection to a divine source. That animal source saved his life and remained with him constantly. **(1)**

Andres also inherited the gift of connecting with the unseen world from his father. The signs began early, in a modern school classroom. For instance, hummingbirds used to land on his desk in his first-grade classroom. Other odd things happened, like a snake appearing in his lunchbox at school! A Raven even pooped on the top of his head in front of all the tribal elders! (1) As it turned out, he and the Raven bonded, and that animal spirit remains with him to this day. He says that he is communicating in one form or another with animal spirits most of the time, and for that reason, his life has never lacked adventure.

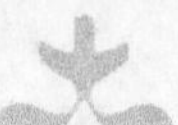

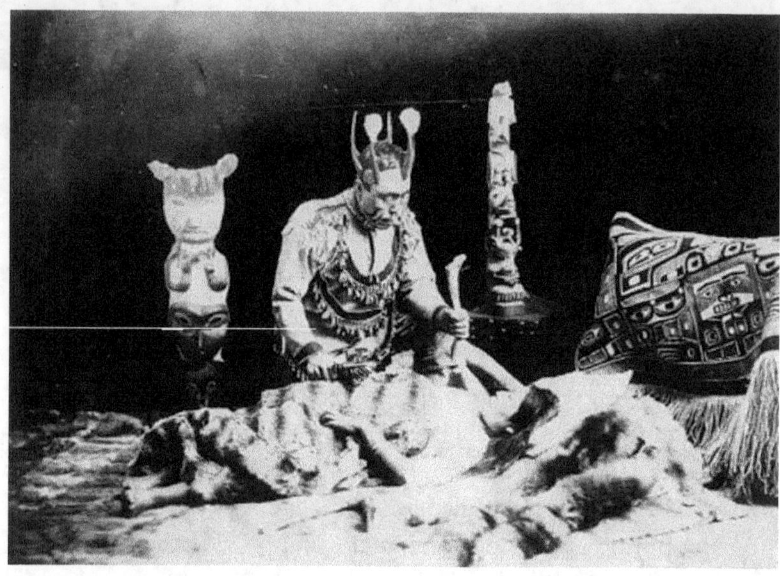

Native shaman, Alaska, circa 1905, Caption written on image: Indian Witch Doctor. Case & Draper. PH Coll 413.Album 16.24c, photographer Case & Draper, photo current location University of Washington: Special Collections

The Medicine Wheel — The Inner Sacred Journey

Sometimes Native Americans referred to the medicine wheel as the sacred hoop. It represented the totality of abundant life, bounty in all forms, knowledge, and wisdom as it showed the four directions, east, west, north, and south. Mainly native tribes used it as a tool to understand themselves and receive support from the unseen world.

Different tribes had different medicine wheels, but the wheel generally was divided into four sections represented by four colors, symbolic of the seasons. The four sections signify east, west, north, and south. Often black, white, red, and yellow are used, yet different tribes use various colors. They placed primary sacred objects like stones or feathers in the center, as well as a picture of the sun or moon. **(5)**

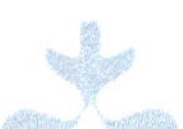

Through prayer and ritual offering, different energies or characteristics are transmitted through the medicinal wheel in a ceremony. **(1)**

East — symbolic rebirth, strength, power of expression, new beginnings
West — creativity, spiritual goals, compassion, imagination, vision, dreams
South — overcoming obstacles, purity, faith, playfulness, protection, change
North — teaching, abundance, gratitude, trust, sacred wisdom, empathy, and intuition

It acted like the medicine bundle in some ways, but it was in a different visual form. Healers and medicine men put feathers, rocks, or other sacred objects on the wheel. They placed medicinal substances on the wheel to call forth their power and offer prayers to anyone suffering and seeking relief from the plant world. Tribal members sometimes decorated the wheel or wore more miniature versions of it that they crafted on their clothing. **(5)**

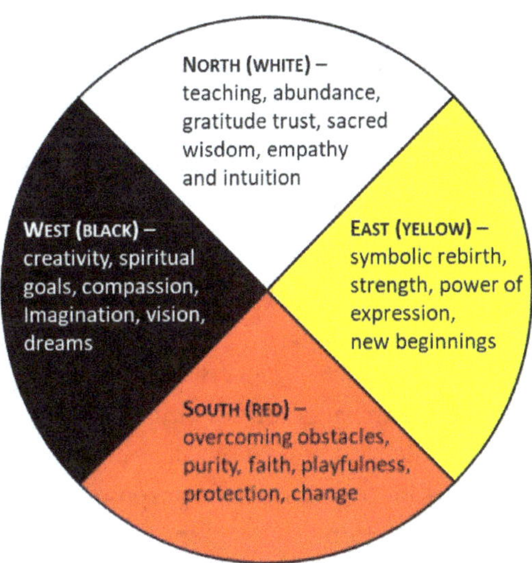

The Native Americans Medicine Wheel also called Sacred Hoop.

4.3   Omens and Symbols

Bobby Lake Thom or Medicine Grizzly Bear is a direct descendent of the Karuk/Seneca tribe. He tells stories about how his ancestors remained safe and protected because they had an acute awareness of signs from nature that exposed them to act or not to work. He relays:

"For years, I wondered how my grandfather knew a flood was coming. Many people were amazed at the so-called psychic premonitions and power he often demonstrated. Whether it is good news or bad news, a favorable situation or a negative situation, for some reason, he always seemed to have a way of knowing before certain events would occur. My great-grandmother, Kitty Hawk, was like that too. She would say that a little bird had foretold something or forewarned her when questioned. **(1)**

Lake Thom describes that his grandparents were trained to see the world differently. Stories shaped his mind. He remembered parts of these stories. As he grew older, he learned more stories. They formed a very rich treasury of guidance for thinking, behaving, believing, interacting, exploring, worshiping, and celebrating.

Native Americans built intuition, awareness, listening, and sacred communication into daily life. The following sections cover the general ways many Native American tribes approached the ordinary day today and the more extraordinary ceremonies and rituals that took place on particular occasions.

There is a *difference between rituals and ceremonies*, although sometimes they are referred to interchangeably. A ritual denotes a collection of actions designed for their value symbolically. A ceremony, by contrast, brought people together for a particular purpose, either seasonally, to celebrate a victory, to call forth ancestral spirits at a specific time, or for another purpose.

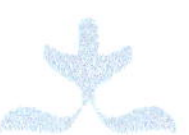

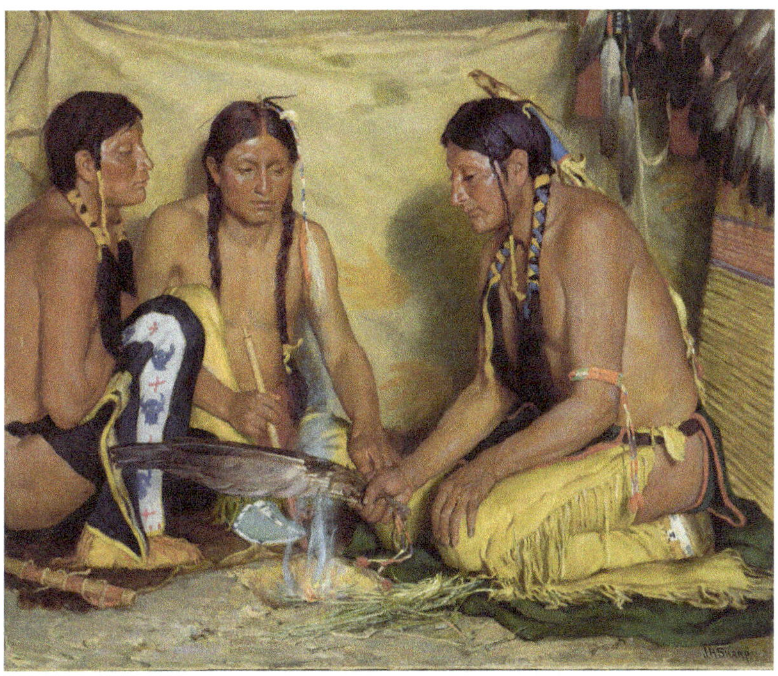

Making Sweet Grass Medicine, Blackfoot Ceremony around 1920, artist Joseph Henry Sharp (1859–1953), Painting oil on canvas, Smithsonian American Art Museum, Cretit to Bequest of Victor Justice Evans

4.4   Ceremony

More ceremonies existed in Native American culture than this section can cover. However, many times these ceremonies contained common elements. The critical thing to understand is the general sequence of events and sacred ceremonial objects. Most rites included prayers, dancing, and chanting, also considered forms of medicine. Dancing and chanting could convey energy, and tribes believed these acts could transform matter.

The four-day Sun Dance of the Buffalo Cow Society

Like many cultures, Native Americans considered sun worship a pivotal practice. Let's look at the four-day Sun Dance held yearly by a female society known as the Buffalo Cow Society within the Matoki tribe of the Plains people. First, the society leader provided a pole to erect a communal tipi where they held the ceremony. The participants lived together during the entire period. They were not allowed to sleep and remained awake the whole time. It isn't easy to think in modern terms about staying awake for four continuous days in a sacred state of worship! By day two, most modern people would take sleeping pills to go back to sleep. Yet a ceremonial situation is quite different.

The participants chose four men who sang and chanted during those days while two other men became attendants to the participants and messengers.

The women wore different costumes. Each head dressing or bonnet they wore carried a particular meaning, snake bonnets, scabby wool bonnets, and buffalo wool or feather bonnets. They danced while blowing on bone whistles.

Participants had often made sacred vows before coming — if not a vow, at least a promise. They offered berry soup, a delicacy, or another type of soup, signifying their shared possession, and used particular prayers to find a resolution. If someone had a specific need, they gave tobacco a prime offering. However, they told the medicine man's leader about their problem when they offered the tobacco. The medicine man would pray to meditate, often entering into a state of altered consciousness. At this time, members petitioned to gain entrance into the society. They brought a horse, gun, property, or other valuable objects.

The ceremony had another element, a jesting or active component. Jest, joking, and playful behavior were also Native American lore and beliefs. A possibility always remained in life that something could appear in disguise, or a surprise in the sacred storyline would create a turn of events. In this case, at night, the men would return home, and some

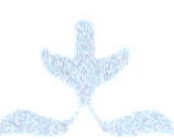

of the women remained at the ceremony, dressed as men, acting out the male roles. During the last phase of the ceremony, women made fake medicine bundles and play-acted like men. Sometimes they even rolled up blankets, pretending like medicine bundles, while acting.

On the fourth day, before sunrise, all participants scouted the plains for the lowest spot they could find. They imitated the buffalo searching for water. When their leader directed them with a particular command, all participants 'became the buffalo' and laid down. Then the senior members made sacrifices, offered presents, and built a sacred fire with cow dung. When participants smelled the smoke, they ran back to the tipi. Female members ran around the tipi in the direction of the sun until the scabby bull bonneted members ceremonially pulled them back to their seats **(2)**

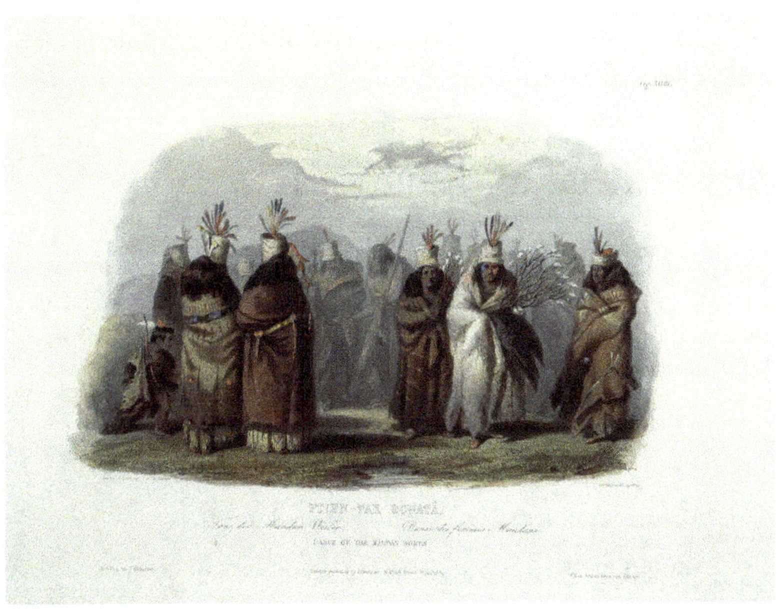

Ptihn-Tak-Ochatä — Dance of the Mandan Women by *Karl Bodmer*, 1840–1843

Death Ceremonies

Because over 562 tribes have existed in the U.S. alone, presenting a standard Native American death ceremony prototype is hard. Heaven and hell as concepts did not exist. Some tribes believed in reincarnation. Spirits could travel after death. They would visit the living and deliver memorable messages.

Sometimes the tribe decorated the body or painted it. Other tribes refused to speak the name of the dead for a year to avoid their spirit revisiting the living and negatively affecting them.

Generally, the tribe placed valuable items near the bodies of the deceased. Some tribes left the body near the water; others put it on a platform. Some constructed funeral pyres. Funerals for children comforted those left behind and carried the child's spirit to a place for evolution and growth. The mother would take some of the child's hair, put it on a doll's head, and carry it with her for a year to assuage her grief. **(6)**

4.5   Ritual and Symbols

Native Americans lived through a series of ritual acts and symbols day by day. Symbols and rituals served as links to activate powers. Even their names, like Red Cloud, Sitting Bull, or Lone Wolf, became symbolic of the power they carried. Performing ritual meant using:

- A drum
- A song
- A religious object like feathers or sacred tree bark
- Various foods
- A pipe is usually called a peace pipe for smoking an offering like tobacco in a communal circle. This practice was quite powerful and taught community members the value of being silent and listening while another tribal member spoke.

Most corn-growing cultures have corn ceremonies and rituals. Corn, cornmeal, and corn pollen commonly symbolized fertility and med-

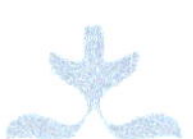

icine. Today many ways are still practiced that use cornmeal or corn pollen. Cornmeal is an accessible offering to learn. One can offer a sacred prayer or blessing in the early morning and leave a small dish of cornmeal as an offering for animals in the front yard. A small amount of cornmeal can be placed near the four corners of a house to call in abundance.

The Navajo used corn pollen in "The Navajo Wind Way" ritual. Pueblo tribes used corn as a ritual object. The Seneca even tell a story about how corn was strong medicine for wound healing:

In many stories, the Corn Woman appears. Sometimes she is killed, or her head is cut off. Her body is flung around, and her blood turns into the earliest corn plants during the spring. Beautiful corn women appear to hunters as long corn stalks to teach them the secrets of capturing their prey. Rituals are performed to summon her and ask for guidance. (2)

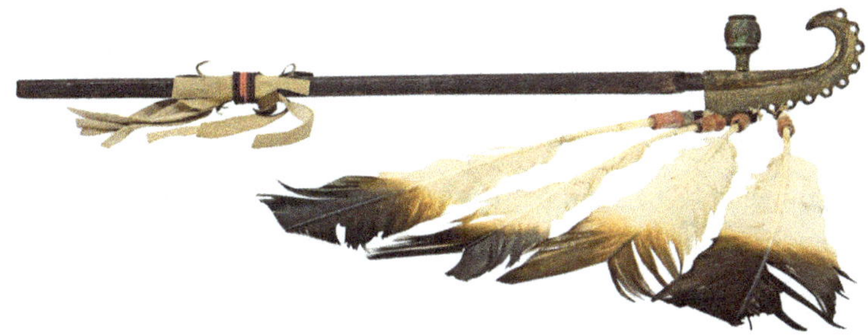

Totems

In the classic book "Animal Speak" by Ted Andrews, he gives readers step-by-step guidelines on connecting with their totem animals. It is a simple process. Even if living in an urban environment, these connections are possible. This elder reminds us that we are born to make these connections. Even before one is aware of an animal totem, those animals have already been aware of you. The following section is taken from his fantastic work. Andrews is adept at helping the newcomer to Native American experience feel at ease. He advises us that:

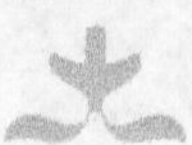

- You accept that every animal has a vital spirit. That soul spirit of the animal is powerful.

- The spirit will communicate messages directly to humans, or another spirit can work through that animal as well.

- Animals have various gifts, skills, and abilities, just like humans.

- The animal is there to develop the call to our power, teach us about medicine, and guide our development to become more effective in all we do.

- Usually, our totem comes from wild animals, not domestic ones. However, there are exceptions on a case-by-case basis if the emotional pull is strong.

- The animal chooses the person and not the other way around. Andrews cautions his readers that people often want to select glamorous animals for their totem. They do not wish to the 'mouse' or the frog as their spiritual companion. However, he says wisely, 'it is better to become influential in mouse medicine as it comes to you rather than eagle medicine which does not come to you. That power is yours. You practice it freely, knowing it was not borrowed from anyone else.' **(1)**

We can see how different Native American medicine is from allopathic medicine, where you get a diagnosis for one symptom and receive a prescription.

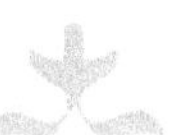

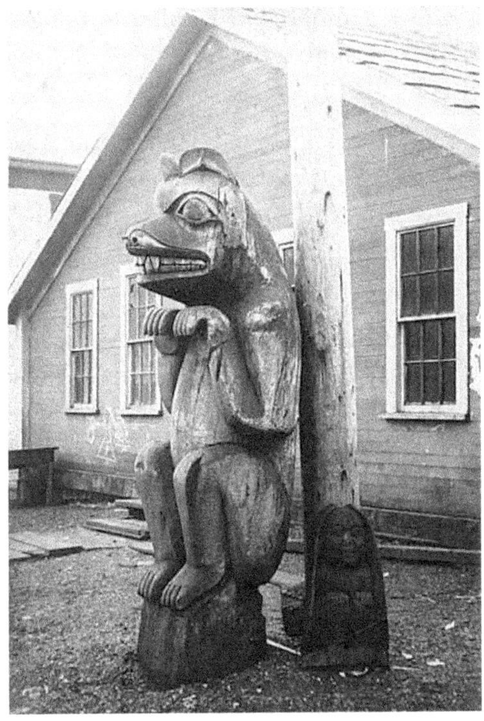

Bear totem, ca 1899, Writing on verso of image: Indian Chief's Bear Totem, Klinquan, Alaska. Photo by B.A. Haldane

Medicine Bundles

Native Americans collected precious, sacred objects and either put them in a handmade bag or wrapped them into a bundle. They called it a medicine bundle. The bundle held a primal and fundamental significance for a tribe. What the tribe had inherited, the powers available to them transferred into their medicinal healing objects and even their identity. Many individuals carried medicine bundles attached to their clothing. Mainly medicine bundles represented an animal or group of animals. The bundles contained bird parts or other animal parts, herbs, feathers, stones, bones, occasionally scalps. One famous medicine bundle story is the 'mountain soil bundle' story of the Blessingway Creation Story. Pawnee tribes relay the powerful details of opening bundles such as the "grain-of-corn bundle" to bring protection and good fortune in the growing season and women who wished to become fertile and bear children. **(2)**

People carefully kept a specific bundle. They maintained it, and they protected it. Tribal members carried the bundles with them when they were buried after death. The community members believed that animals spirits or totems represented in the bundle would come at the time of death to transport the soul to the heavenly realms.

Many tribes held certain herbs in protective and sacred ways. Tobacco was probably considered the holiest herb throughout all tribes (although today it is not utilized in a sacred manner by most people). Most medicine bundles contained tobacco. Sage was perhaps the second most used herb ceremonially, and then accounts vary, but Thyme and Lemon Balm were indeed prized substances. Most people reading this book could grow these same herbs in their kitchen or backyard. Perhaps they are already in your home.

Tobacco bears special consideration for its multiple religious and ceremonial purposes. Many tribes smoked tobacco or put the unsmoked leaves in unique places to aid spirits, animals, and plants. differently

The Seminole Indians gave thanks using tobacco offerings when they avoided danger. They offered the same so that storms and lightning would subside while the Menominee arranged tobacco leaves on the graves of loved ones. Medicinally, tobacco had curative properties. The Iroquois used it to assist with toothaches. For the Cherokee, tobacco leaves could be fried and mixed with other herbs and oil to create a salve for healing the skin. (2)

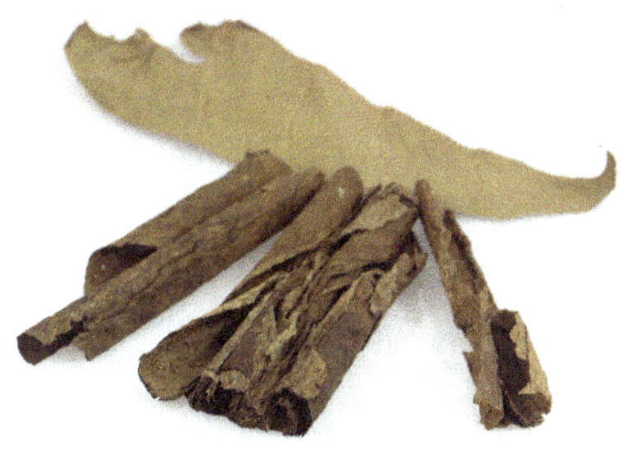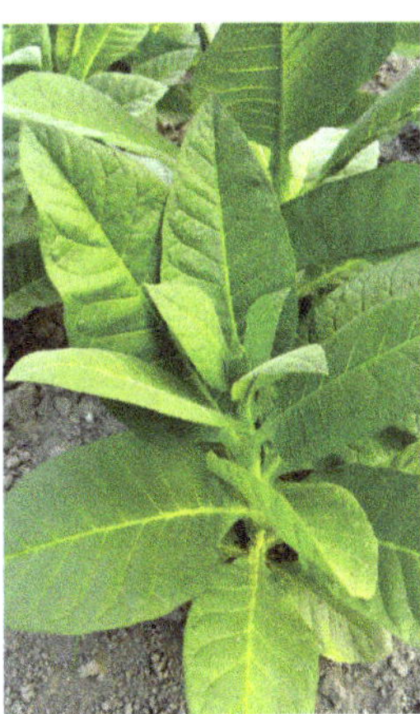

The sacred herb tobacco is dried and processed

Smudging

Smudging was essential practice for releasing negativity, purification, and for blessing. For the budding herbalist, it may be one of the most accessible practices to perform. Native Americans would typically dry stalks of the herbs, cut them, and bind them together into a small bunch. One end of the bunch is lit, just like an incense stick. The practitioner slowly waves the smoke over an individual or throughout the four corners of a room, chanting. The primary purpose is to clear stagnant energy and usher in feelings of peace and harmony. Sometimes a healer would perform this act with tobacco. Inside the home, it wasn't uncommon for a female to perform this ritual as needed.

Sage — All types of Sage signify wisdom, strength, and clarity. Sage supports maternal and female power.

Cedar — Cedar is a powerful cleanser of negativity. It could balance an imbalanced setting, mainly if evil spirits were present. Cedar connects people to a spiritual world and at the same time reconnects humans to each other.

Sweetgrass — Sweetgrass figured prominently in most Native American tribes as a vehicle to send prayers to the spirit world. The herb resembles hair and became known as the hair of the earth itself. Tribal members felt that the herb carries a holy breath within it that transported their prayers to the world beyond.

Other traditional possibilities are Mugwort, Birch, Juniper Berry, Peppermint, Wormwood, Thyme, Lemon Balm. We will explore these herbs later in the Materia Medica section and build your apothecary.

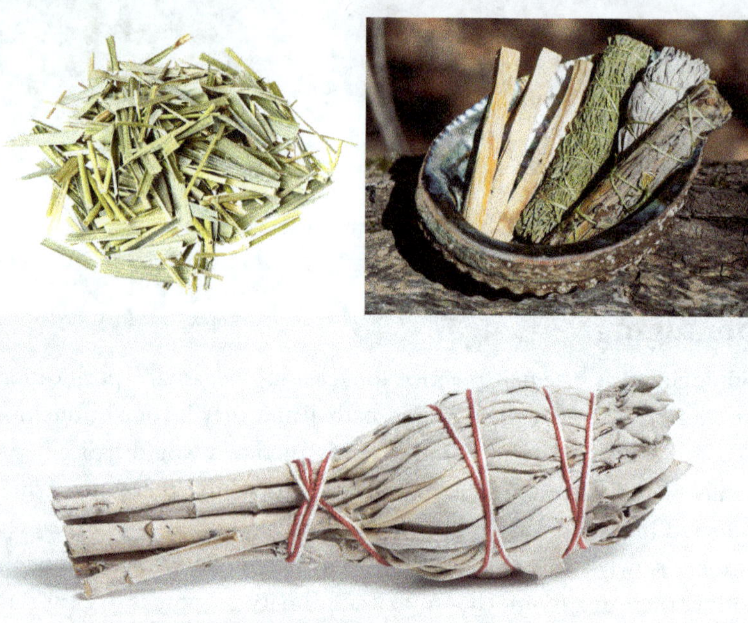

Smudge Kits — Top picture f.l.t.r: Dried Palo Santo sticks,
Cedar, Sage and Mugwort in an Abalone shell.
Lower picture: White Sage Smudge Stick

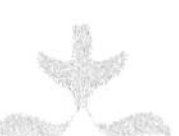

Sources

(1)   Andrews, Ted, Animal Speak: The Spiritual and Magical Powers of Creatures Great and Small, Minnesota: Llewellyn Publications, 2000. pp.17-24, 50, 108

(2)   Gill, Sam D. and Irene F. Sullivan, Dictionary of Native American Mythology, New York: Oxford University Press, 1992. p. 238,

(3)   Lake Thom, Bobby, A Guide to Native American Nature Symbols, Stories and Ceremonies, New York: Penguin Books, 1997.

(4)   Native American Spirituality — Native American Spirituality and Religion (learnreligions.com)

(5)   National Park Service, The Medicine Wheel (U.S. National Park Service) (nps.gov,) updated October 10, 2020

(6)   Funeral Guide, "Death Around the World: Native American Beliefs," *https://www.funeralguide.com/blog/death-around-world*, revised October 14, 2016.

(7)   Philip, Neil, ed., "In A Sacred Manner I Live," New York, Clarion Books, 1997., p. 34

(8)   Public Law 95-341 95th Congress, "American Indian Religious Freedom Act, 1978. STATUTE-92-Pg469.pdf (govinfo.gov)

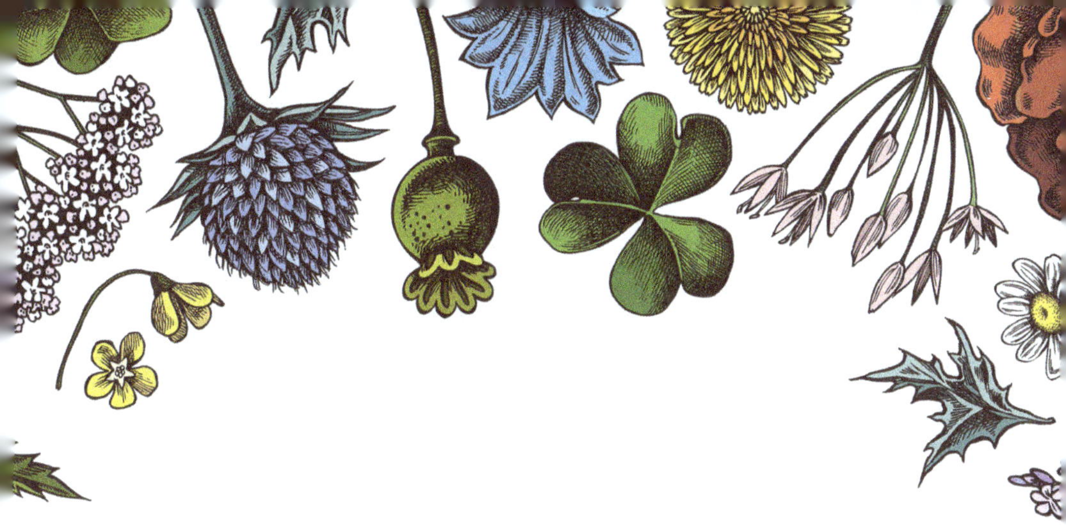

BOOK 2: THE MEDICINE CHEST OF NATIVE AMERICAN TRIBES

"In the old days when we were a strong and happy people, all our power came to us from the sacred hoop of the nation, and so long as the hoop was unbroken, the people flourished. The flowering tree was the living center of the hoop, and the circle of the four quarters nourished it."

—BLACK ELK (7)

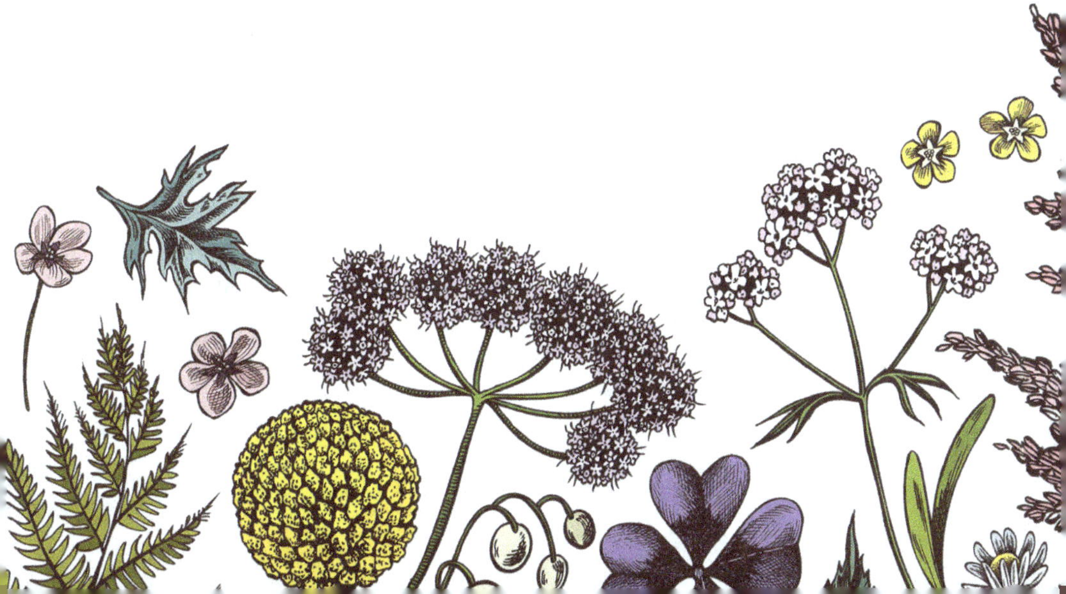

5   Native American Herbal Wisdom for Modern Times

The following section will answer the most common questions about working with herbs. Answering your questions and providing resources at this stage will assist your preparatory phase in creating a user-friendly apothecary. This session contains time-tested herbal wisdom tailored for the modern herbal seeker.

5.1   How do Herbal Medicine and Conventional Medicine Differ?

1. Conventional medicine treats symptoms and diseases. It has existed for about 150 years. On the other hand, Traditional medicine includes integrative approaches used for thousands of years.

2. Conventional medicine treats symptoms separately from the whole person. Traditional medicine integrates all treatments holistically to improve the body, mind, and spirit.

Herbs contain hundreds and even thousands of phytochemicals or interrelated active compounds. Pharmaceutical manufacturers isolate one substance to act on a particular symptom. Herbalists utilize the whole herb and allow it to have a comprehensive effect on multiple systems in the body.

1. Herbal medicine is typically much less expensive than conventional medical treatments.

2. Pharmaceutical drugs are often hard for the body to process. In the end, side effects may result, creating another condition as problematic as the original one.

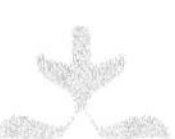

3. Herbal medicine can simultaneously provide prevention, nutrition, symptom management, stress management, and contribute to longevity. Conventional medicine provider a singular cure.

Ideally, any medicine incorporates all tools and wisdom that help the person achieve balance, optimize all systems and prevent illness whenever possible. The National Center for Complementary and Alternative Medicine (NCCAM) recognizes the Native American (N.A.) healing system as a comprehensive, holistic system for a wide range of chronic and acute illnesses.

Many Native Americans and their traditional medical healers combine their traditional practices with conventional medicine (3). Cooperation is required from both medical perspectives to serve the whole person, not just a part of the person. Surgical procedures, for instance, such as correcting cataracts or medical interventions such as chemotherapy and radiation are essential. However, traditional medicine can help with pain from the surgery, the stress of recovery, or digestive issues when the patient is bedridden.

Robert Gallegos is a traditional Native American healer. He explains the core of his self-healing journey when faced with an accident that shattered the bones in one of his legs, began with visualizing himself as a whole. Second, his recovery was based on his connection to what he calls 'the Great Creator', and to all of the elements. Third, he utilized sacred objects, herbs, rituals and prayer.

Gallegos gives us his prescription for healing. A person cannot heal if they are worried, fearful, or frustrated. People have to eat well, exercise, pray and live a balanced life. A healer can only do so much. Then, it is up to the person to heal themselves. All of us have the power to heal ourselves. One of his favorite practices with those he heals is to ask: Can you blink your eyes? Can you wiggle your toes? Of course, people usually nod affirmatively. He tells them, "Everything from your head to your toes belongs to you because you used your muscles, your nerves, your blood, and your skin to wiggle your toes." So, everything in between your head and your toes is under your control.

Confidence in interconnectedness and rising above fear and negativity is the key. He advises people to sit in a calm place, focus on where they are hurting, and visualize a healthy area instead of one that is hurt. From that place, healing ceremonies using sacred objects, and herbs can begin. To this day, using these methods, doctors are astonished that Gallegos was able to heal himself without surgical intervention.

The traditional healer implores people to please find peace, and happiness because true healing becomes impossible if one is stressed out.[1]

5.2   What Are the Main Precautions to Take When Using Herbs?

1. In terms of safety, it is wise to stay informed and cautious about the biased information on herbs. To date, 80% of the worlds' population uses herbs for some portion of their physical care. By 2015 the global herb market reached 100 billion yearly world-wide **(3).**

2. Herbal medicine is a drug and is not free from toxicity and side effects. One has to become aware of what one might feel when taking an herb. One possibility, for instance, is that an herb will initiate a release of toxins from the body. It creates flu-like symptoms.

3. When taking herbs, one must drink water throughout the day. An herb has to move and perform its actions *through the water*. Think of it this way. Your body is approximately 75% water. When any system has an imbalance, water is required to flush any unwanted substance from the body. Herbs create movement in various systems; water is their companion for achieving the desired result. **(4)**

---

[1]   Please see: Gallegos, Robert, "A Native American Traditional Healer Teaches About Self-Healing", June 18, 2017, Native American Traditional Healer teaching about self-healing — YouTube, Seen on February 20, 2022.

4. According to the master herbalist and teacher Michael Tierra, L.Ac, one should note. O.M.D. that Westerners unfamiliar with herbal medical systems tend to take too little of an herb, conclude that herbs are not effective as a result, and discard the treatment (4). Therefore, please review the dosage section in this book carefully.

5. Know the toxicity of an herb, discuss it with a practitioner, and proceed. Awareness and research are the keys. Bear in mind that many herbs can treat a particular issue. There is no reason to use an herb with contraindications if you feel unsafe. Options exist. Well-trained practitioners understand the options and can guide you.

6. Some herbs are more toxic than others. This book avoids those herbs to make the beginner's path more accessible.

7. One must use the right herb for the proper condition. Never think that an herb used to treat asthma will put you to sleep or reduce inflammation. Carefully reading the Materia Medica sections will allow you to match the herb to the ailment.

6   Where can I get herbs, and how are they stored?

Surprisingly it does not take much effort to collect essential herbs. One, you can easily purchase kitchen herbs from any grocery store. Two, you can grow some herbs in pots in your own home, particularly if you do not have garden space. Three, you can grow herbs in your garden. Last but certainly not least, you can forage your own.

6.1   Foraging Herbs

You will be astonished at how many herbs you can find in a small area (approximately ½ acre) that are edible food sources and medicinal as well. Please read the following before you begin gathering herbs:

1. Protect yourself from ticks and any insect or creature by being fully clothed. White cotton clothing is best. It will breathe and make insects visible. Ticks especially do not like white! Wear socks and shoes, not sandals.

2. Cover your clothing with either natural sprays that deter insect ticks or spray your clothing with something more substantial like Permethrin.

3. Lyme's Disease from ticks is also something you want to avoid at all costs. After you come indoors from foraging, immediately change your clothes and take a shower, checking every single area of the body. Again when you dry off, check for ticks, and then a third time as you get dressed, check for ticks.

In addition to protection from insects:

1. Bring a basket, a small shopping bag, and other smaller bags to separate the herbs when you find them.

2. Native American protocols tell us to pick only a third of that herb when you find an herb. Consequently, the other ⅔ will thrive, grow, and remain available for others.

3. Prepare an area to dry your herbs. For instance, if you are harvesting Mint and acquiring several branches, you can tie the stems and hang them upside down. When you gather individual leaves, roots, or flowers, you can cut open a paper bag, spread it across a flat surface that is not in the sunlight, and dry your herbs there. Parchment paper works well also. Drying times vary. In the case of Yarrow, it is a dry leafy herb, so it will not take much time to dry. However, holds more Mullein leaves hold more water and take longer to dry.

Not all open land or public land is suitable for foraging. Always check before you forage to ensure that the property owner permits gathering there. For this reason, I strongly recommend starting in your backyard first. The Native American Indians believe that the appropriate herb you need for healing yourself grows *within 50 feet* of where you live for most conditions. It is as if the plant world responds to your needs before you even have them — Incredible! Over time this observation has certainly proven true in the lives of many herbalists.

6.2 Purchasing Bulk Herbs and Herbal Formulas

There are a few guidelines to follow when ordering herbs. Generally, you will need one to four ounces of an herb for non-commercial use. Four ounces is more appropriate for a larger family.

Always make sure that:

1. You choose a reputable herb company.

2. Your herbs have color. An herb that is not vibrant will not contain maximum healing qualities.

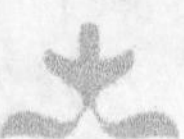

3. Your herbs smell. Many herbs have offensive odors. However, if an herb smells, it contains vitality.

4. They must have a taste. Perhaps the herbs may not always taste great. Many herbs (truthfully the best ones for you) often taste bitter or pungent. Yet the distinctive flavor of the herb is significant. It tells you what qualities of the herb work with which parts of the body. However, this is a more advanced concept that you can explore further in your studies.

5. Your herb should have a direct result. If it does not work:

   - It may not be fresh.

   - It may be the wrong herb.

   - It may take longer to take effect.

   - You may be taking the wrong dosage.

Check with a practitioner to see what is causing the problem.

7   The Actions of Herbs

7.1   Explanation of action words

Understanding herbs and their actions is essential. If you think back to the beginning of the book, we covered the differences between conventional medicine and traditional medicine. When the whole herb is used rather than its component, your body responds holistically. You will be amazed at how many things herbs can do. It is truly a wonder.

If you are already taking medication, you must consult with a trustworthy trained practitioner before taking any herb.

Adaptogens — These help various systems in the body 'adapt' to stress. Adaptogens protect, restore and strengthen. In many cases, they provide nourishment, just like food. This book includes Rosemary, Saw Palmetto, Nettle, Chamomile, Mushrooms (edible ones only), Elderberry, Lemon Balm, Devil's Club, and Ginseng.

Alterative — Provides nourishment and strength for the body via removing toxic metabolic wastes (often from the liver). This book includes Echinacea, Dandelion, Black Cohosh, Yerba Santa, and Red Clover.

Anaesthetic — Depresses nerve function, thereby creating a loss of sensation or consciousness. This book only deals with topical anesthetics. Examples from this book include Plantain, Oak, and White Willow Bark.

Anthelmintic — Destroy worms and parasites in the digestive tract — Examples from this book include: Mugwort and Black Gum Bark

Antiemetic — Will reduce nausea and help prevent vomiting. This book includes Ginger, Meadowsweet, Mint, and Black Gum Bark.

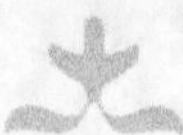

Anti-Lithic — These herbs prevent gravel or stones in the urinary system. Examples from this book include Uva Ursi, Saw Palmetto, and Blackberry.

Anti-inflammatory — These work directly on tissues to soothe. They do not interrupt the practical aspects of natural inflammatory reaction, but they reduce the harmful effects of inflammation. This book includes Chamomile, Ginger, Lemon Balm, Meadowsweet, Rosemary, Goldenrod, Arnica, Sage, and White Willow Bark.

Antispasmodic — This eases muscle cramping, as well as muscular tension. Antispasmodics include nervines that reduce psychological and physical stress (the brilliant design of nature!) Some antispasmodics lessen muscle spasms throughout the body, while others work with specific organs or systems. This book includes Ginger, Black Cohosh, Lemon Balm, Mint, California Poppy, and Sage.

Antitussive — This category prevents coughs, both wet and dry. This book includes Butterfly Weed, Boneset, Ginger, and Mullein.

Antiviral — Prohibits the actions of a virus. This book includes Elderberry, Devil's Club, Milkweed flowers, and Ginger.

Astringent — Astringents act to dry out a cell; they squeeze excess fluid from cells and carry unwanted substances out of the body. Astringents bind to mucous membranes. *Mucous membranes are the carrier of bacteria and the seeds of illness.* Astringents also break up fats and tighten tissues, releasing toxins. They assist with weight loss. They help break down proteins, reduce irritation and inflammation, and decrease fluid loss. Examples in this book include Yarrow, Uva Ursi, Rosehips, Blackberry leaves, and Oak Bark.

Bitter — These are exceptional herbs that have profound benefits. A bitter herb sends a message to the gut via the central nervous system. It tells the gut to release digestive hormones that stimulate the appetite, give rise to the flow of digestive juices and then increase bile flow. Consequently, the liver receives the signal to work more effectively with bile to detoxify and repair the gut. This book includes Dandelion, Dock, Echinacea, Nettle, Red Clover, Yarrow, and Yerba Santa.

Most dark leafy greens are also bitter. They are medicine in and of themselves. Befriend your bitter herbs wholeheartedly. Even though this category of herbs tastes bitter, remember that they clean the liver. The liver executes over 400 different functions. Three essential functions are blood filtration, metabolic stability, and nutrient synthesis. Hardly a person exists who does not need to optimize liver function.

Carminative — Carminatives are rich in aromatic oils. They stimulate proper digestion, soothe irritations along the intestinal wall, reduce inflammation in general, help alleviate gas and promote easy elimination. This book includes Chamomile, Ginger, Dandelion, Lemon Balm, and Mint.

Cardiotonic — A beneficial herb that increases the strength and tone of the heart. Examples from this book include Milkweed, Ginger, and Yarrow.

Diaphoretic — Opens channels to detoxify and increase perspiration. In the case of bronchitis or chest tightness, it opens the lungs and initiates detoxification. This book includes Mint, Butterfly Weed, Boneset, Goldenrod, and Yerba Santa.

Emetic — It causes vomiting: Examples from this book include Boneset.

Emollient — Applied to the skin to protect, soften and soothe — Examples from this book include: Plantain (soothes both internally and externally), Oatstraw (soothes both internally and externally)

Expectorant: An expectorant removes mucous or other unwanted substances. This book includes Butterfly Weed, Yerba Santa, Ginger, and Boneset.

Febrifuge — This lowers a fever. Examples from this book include Boneset and Yarrow.

Galactagogue — Increases breast milk flow in nursing mothers. Examples from this book include: Nettle (or its cousin Blessed Thistle), Ginger (or Fenugreek seed if you have it on hand).

(California poppy or a simple tea made from fresh parsley can dry up breast milk — the opposite action.)

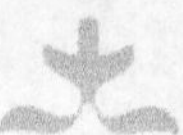

Hepatics — Hepatics tone and strengthen the liver and increase bile flow. Examples from this book include Dandelion, Echinacea, and Red Clover.

Hypotensive — This lowers blood pressure. Examples from this book include Ginger and Nettle.

Laxatives — Laxatives stimulate bowel movements. Proper elimination is the cornerstone of good health. We should not have to rely on laxatives all the time to optimize digestive function. However, they keep us out of trouble until we address our deeper issues. We should consider all aspects of our diet instead of becoming too reliant on laxatives. This book includes Chamomile, Dandelion, and Dock (Yellow).

Nervines — Nervines tone the nervous system and are restorative. They are either nervous tonics that strengthen and restore, nervous relaxants that ease anxiety in the mind and body, or nerve stimulants that work directly on neural activity. This book includes Chamomile, Sage, Hops, Lemon Balm, Rose, and California Poppy.

Oxytocic — Stimulates uterine contractions and assists in childbirth — Examples from this book include: Black Cohosh, Nettle, Sage, Mugwort, Rosemary, and Yarrow. ***(On the other hand, if you do not want to stimulate uterine contractions, avoid these herbs.)***

Rubefacient — Dilates the capillaries and increases circulation in the skin. It draws blood from deeper areas of the body to the skin surface. Examples from this book include Rosemary and Ginger.

Sedative — Calms the nerves. Release stress and nervousness from the body. This book includes California Poppy, Hops, Sage, and White Willow Bark.

Stimulant — Increases speed of physiological functions. Examples from this book include Ginseng, Ginger, Peppermint, and Rosemary.

Styptic — Stops or reduces external bleeding by containing concentrated astringents. Examples from this book include Yarrow, Plantain, and Cattails.

Tonic herbs strengthen and revitalize a particular organ system or the entire body. This book includes Acorns, Blackberries, Ginger, Boneset,

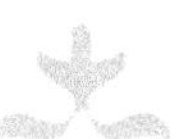

Dandelion, Green Brier, Horsetail, Pine, Nettle, Saw Palmetto, Rosehips, and Uva Ursi.

Vermifuge — Rids the intestines of worms. Examples from this book include: Mugwort, Black Gum Bark (and as an aside, the simple kitchen herb Garlic)

Vulnerary — Contains properties that heal wounds. This book includes Plantain, Boneset, Cattail, Horsetail, Mullein, Yarrow, Yerba Santa, and Black Gum Bark.

Knowing how herbs behave allows one to use them more confidently. Also, it helps you understand the herbs you will use most frequently.

7.2 The effects of taste and temperature

When you go further in your herbal studies, you will learn more about other herbal properties such as *temperature* (e.g., hot, cold) and *taste* (e.g., bitter, pungent, sour, sweet). Ancient medical systems such as Ayurveda and Traditional Chinese medicine used a model of different constitutional types that matched herbs to an individual constitution. They are added in the Materia Medica to provide a complete profile also to the more advanced herbalist.

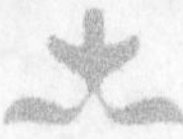

Sources

(1)   American Herbalists Guild, Herbal Medicine F.A.Q.s | American Herbalists Guild, Seen: January 21, 2020

(2)   Gladstar, Rosemary "The Science and Art of Herbalism," Lesson 1, pp. 6-7, Vermont: Sage Mountain Press, 2014.

(3)   Koithan, M., & Farrell, C. (2010). Indigenous Native American Healing Traditions. The journal for nurse practitioners: J.N.P., 6(6), 477–478. *https://doi.org/10.1016/j.nurpra.2010.03.016*

(4)   Tierra, Michael, L.Ac. O.M.D., "The Way of Herbs," New York: Pocket Books, 1998.

(5)   Zhang, Junhua, et al., "The Safety of Herbal Medicine: From Prejudice to Evidence" Evidence-Based Complementary and Alternative Medicine, Hindawi Publishing Corporation, Volume 2015 |Article ID 316706 | *https://doi.org/10.1155/2015/316706*

8   The Medicine Chest of Native American Tribes

8.1   Why Is Materia Medica Important?

Every herbalist learns about herbs by studying Materia Medica. Materia Medica is the history of the collected knowledge about the therapeutic properties of any substance used for healing. Cultures have orally transmitted, or collected and written down, Materia Medica for thousands of years. Their firsthand knowledge of many herbs is currently verified by scientific studies. Chamomile and Ginseng uses for instance are backed by substantial research.

This section introduces the concept of Standard Dosages using the different preparation options. A Standard Dose refers to the amount of an herb that typically alleviates a chronic condition. Please refer to the Dosage section and read it carefully. Always remember that ultimately every individual is different. Each body has it's own way of responding to any medicine, no matter what type it is or what dose is given.

Materia Medica usually contains the following classifications:

1. Common name of the herb

2. Latin name of the herb or herb species

3. Actions — meaning what an herb does

4. Common usage — sometimes called Indications. It suggests main herbal uses.

5. Preparation and dosage — meaning proper herbal ingestion

6. Contraindications — meaning reasons not to consume an herb, or precautions.

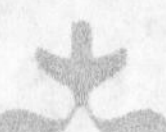

7. Careful study of these categories, makes a competent and knowledgeable herbalist. Continuing observation of the plant world, learning about illnesses, and over time matching the correct remedy to the person will ensure competency.

8. Checking with an herbal teacher or practitioner will help tremendously.

9. Finally, have confidence in your ability to connect to and respect the wisdom of nature, as Native Americans.

8.2   My choice of 40 Native American Healing Herbs

For the beginner, choosing herbs is often a bewildering process. This section will help you streamline your choices. Always remember that one herb can do many things. So, the following list includes many full-spectrum herbs. Many Master Herbalists teach that using fewer herbs more wisely is better.

The following herbs are Native American healing substances chosen for the following reasons:

1. They are sustainable, meaning that they are produced wisely, in order to avoid endangerment to the survival of the plant.

2. They are either easy to buy or to forage.

3. Many are suitable for vulnerable populations like children and seniors.

4. A good number of them alleviate cold, cough, bronchial distress, and flu which comprise the most common ailments.

5. A large portion of them are 'adaptogenic' and help the body adapt to various forms of stress.

Research has repeatedly shown that one must first diminish stress levels when working with any imbalance. Many herbs treat symptoms and entire systems, provide critical nutrients, *and reduce stress.* These are

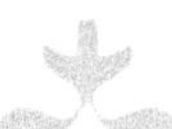

called either primary or secondary adaptogens. Adaptogenic refers to an herbal action. It is essential to learn about Adaptogenic herbs in today's world because they will be your trustworthy companions throughout life. In the Actions section, many herbs are 'adaptogenic.' These substances are an invaluable resource for strength and restoration.

Many plants have similar actions. Whenever applicable these similarities are discussed. It will help you understand ways to use different herbs for the same condition.

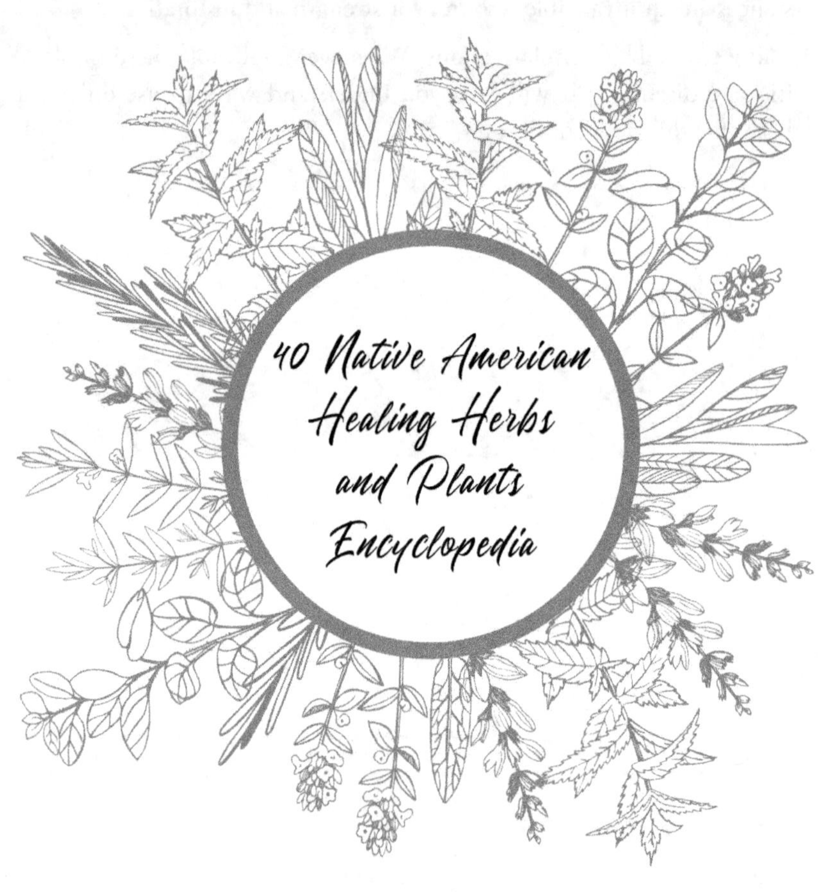
40 Native American
Healing Herbs
and Plants
Encyclopedia

#1 – Arnica

Arnica Montana, sources (18) (5)

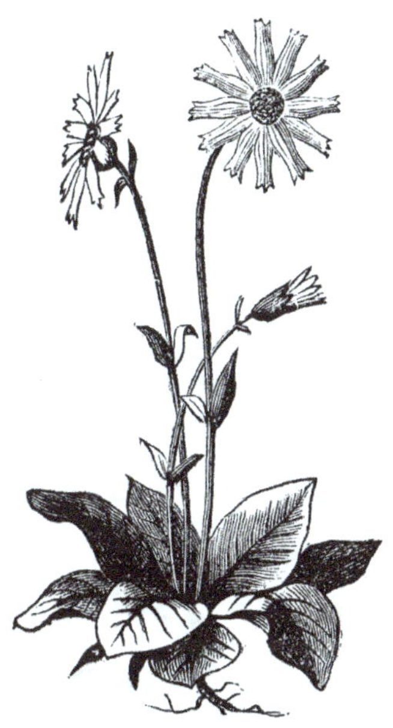

Edible Part Used: flower heads

Actions: anti-inflammatory, vulner-ary

Preparation and Dosage: Topical dosage of a liniment, cream or gel, or a compress from the flowers every 4 hours for chronic pain (e.g., os-teoarthritis) and every two to three hours for acute pain (e.g. Following, surgery)

Contraindications: THIS HERB IS POISONOUS. DO NOT INGEST IT UNLESS YOU TAKE IT AS A CERTIFIED HOMOEOPATHIC REMEDY FROM A CERTIFIED PRACTITIONER

Habitat: Arnica grows in meadows or clay soils in upper elevations (9,800 ft./3000 m) It does not thrive in colder regions and is more common in Central to Northwest Mountain regions.

Common uses: Arnica, when ingested, can be poisonous. However, it is a superior herb used topically for bruises and sprains. Those familiar with Arnica carry a vial of the homeopathic remedy if they fall or get a bruise. Follow the directions. It is easy to dispense and also indispensable!

As long as the skin is not broken, you can use Arnica topically for muscular rheumatic pain, arthritis, or inflammation.

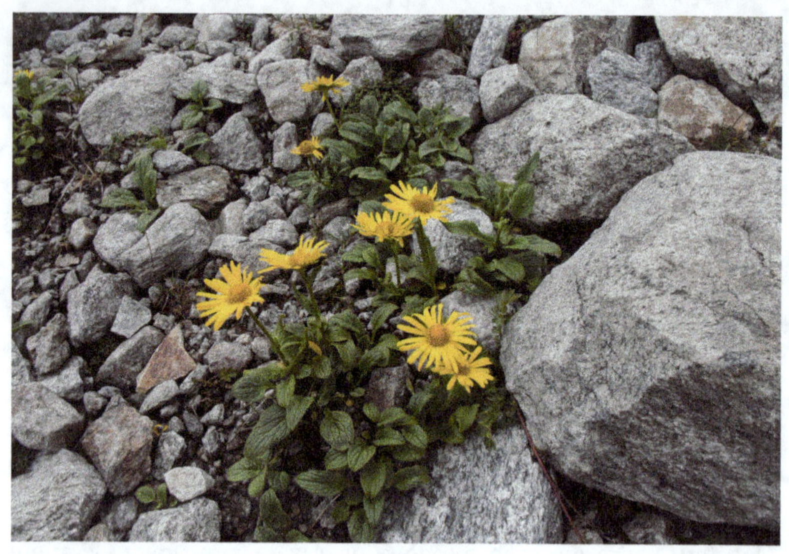

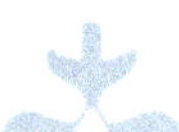

#2 – Blackberry

Rubus Fruticosus, sources: (3) (9) (17) (18)

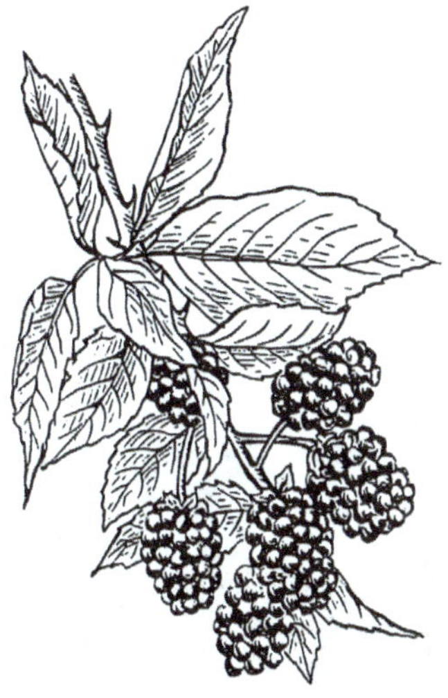

Parts Used: Berries, leaves, roots, and bark.

Taste: Berries are sweet, leaves and bark are astringent and cooling.

Actions: Berries are tonic, leaves and root bark are antipyretic, astringent, and hemostatic.

Preparation and Dosage: Standard tea dosage applies. Take one teaspoon of the dried leaves or root in boiling water. Infuse the leaves, decoct the roots. Take one cup of either leaf or root tea three times daily.

Contraindications: Please follow the recommended dosage.

Habitat: Blackberries still grow in the wild. They thrive in part sun and partly shady areas with just the right amount of rain. Always check and make sure you are eating the right berry in the wilderness. Take it home first if you are unsure, and check it using photos from a reliable source.

Common uses: Blackberries are good for anemia and also blood sugar stabilization. It is important to remember that most berries strengthen kidney and adrenal function. Native tribes understood how powerful berries were. Soups made from berries or dried berries made an ideal ceremonial offering.

Berries were a common and primary tribal medicine throughout the Northeast and the Northwest. Healers used the leaves for fevers, colds, sore throats, and vaginal discharge. The root and stem bark treated diarrhea and dysentery.

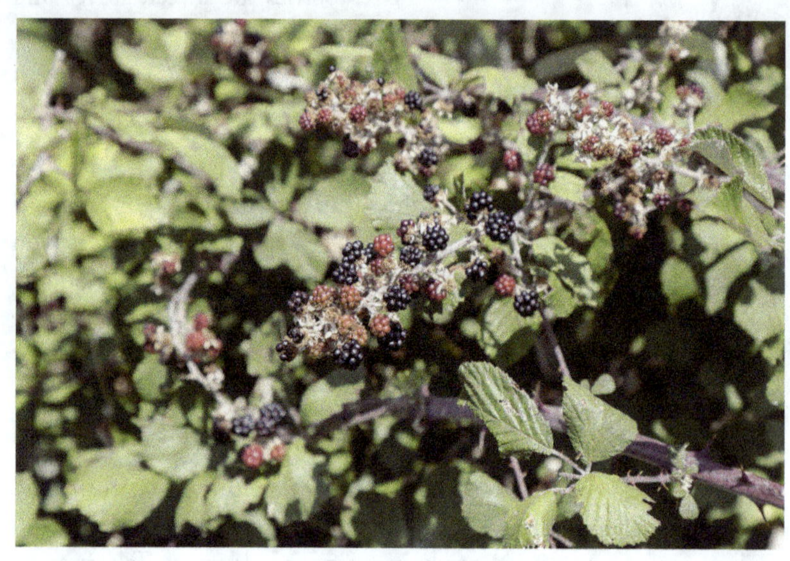

#3 – Black Cohosh

Chimicifuga Racemose, sources: (11) (21)

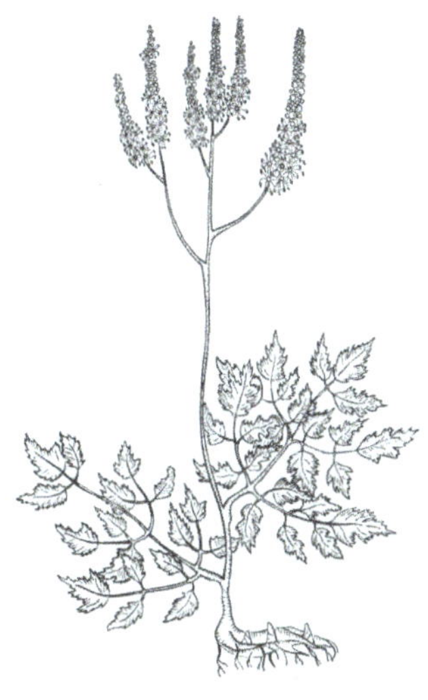

Parts Used: Root

Taste: sweet, pungent, slightly bitter, cool

Actions: antispasmodic, expectorant, emmenagogue, diaphoretic, alterative

Preparation and Dosage: Standard tea dosage applies. Take one teaspoon of the dried root in one cup of boiling water three times daily.

Contraindications: Please follow the recommended dosage.

Habitat: Black Cohosh grows in shade to part shade. Sometimes it does thrive in full sun, but it always prefers rich, moist soil. The flowers are white, spikes with multiple buds. It is more common in all Northern climates.

Common uses: Most Northern tribes used this herb, especially for healing gynecological issues. Black cohosh works for most nervous conditions. It relieves nerve pains and neuralgia in general. Also, it subdues the pains of childbirth and stimulates menstrual flow when it has stalled. Interestingly, it soothes asthma and coughs.

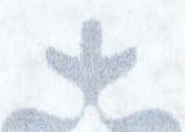

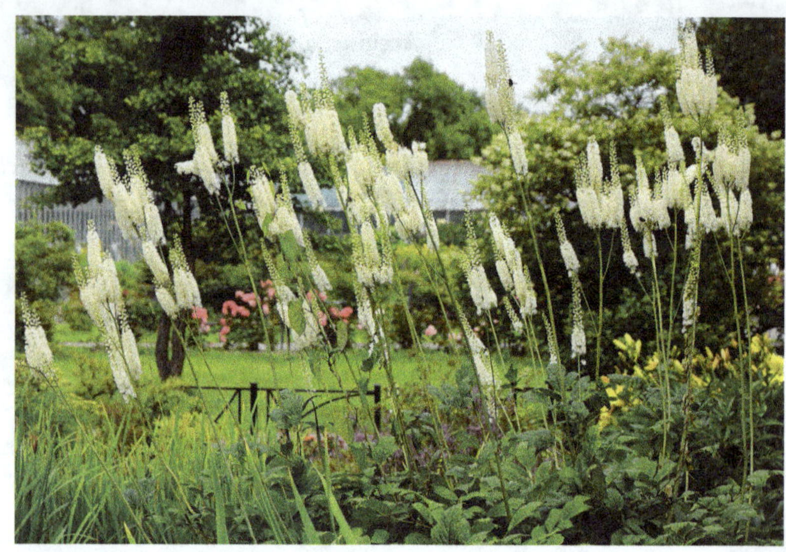

#4 – Black Gum Bark

Nissa Sylvatica, sources: (13)

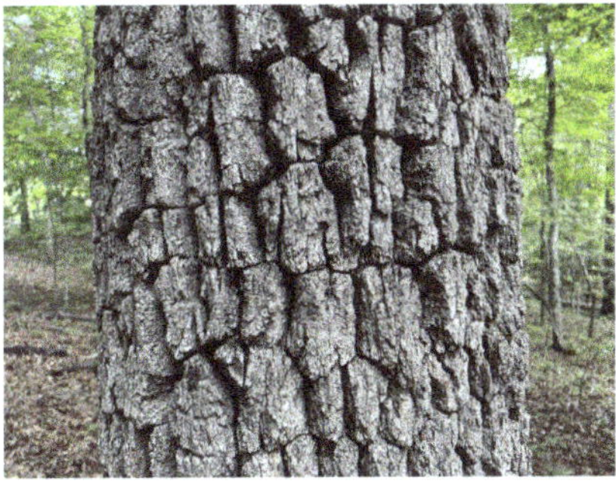

Black Gum Tupeolo tree bark (top) and autumn picture (bottom)

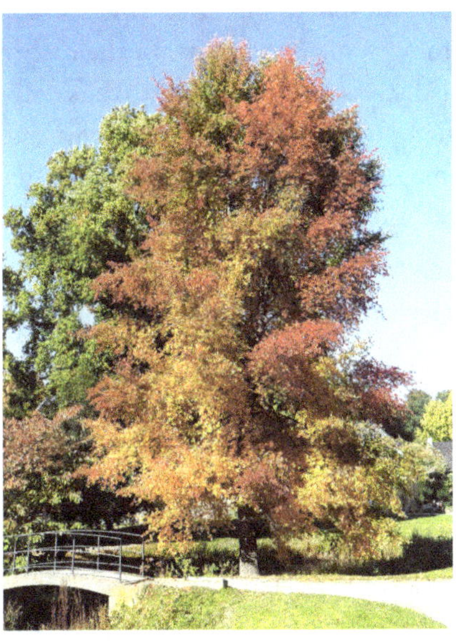

Parts Used: Both outer and inner bark, roots.

Taste: bitter.

Actions: anthelmintic, antiemetic, vulnerary.

Preparation and Dosage: Standard tea dosage applies. Take one teaspoon of the dried bark or root in one cup of boiling water three times daily.

Contraindications: Please follow the recommended dosage.

Habitat: Black Tupelo grows from southwestern Maine to New York in the uplands, in stream bottoms.

Common uses: The Cherokee tribes used Black Tupelo. They would fix a bath for children using a decoction of the outer bark for parasites, worms, and diarrhea. The inner bark stopped vomiting. Juice from the roots aided eye infections. A poultice from the bark treated severe infections and wounds, like those from a gunshot. Black Tupelo bark aids childbirth and can prevent hemorrhaging.

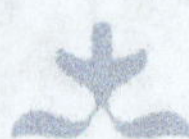

#5 – Boneset

Eupatorium Perfoliatum, sources: (6) (11)

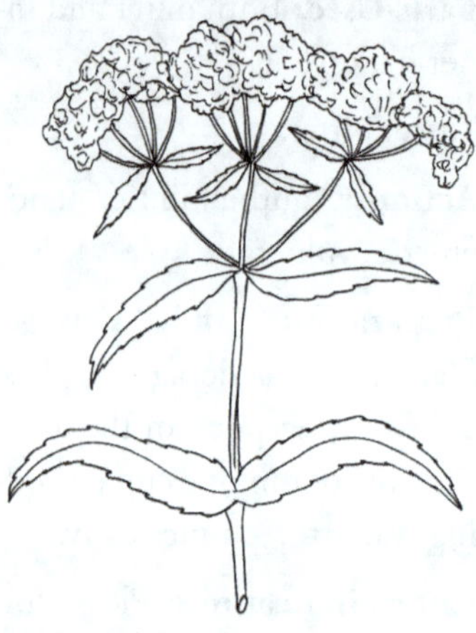

Parts Used: dried aerial parts.

Taste: very bitter

Actions: diaphoretic, laxative, tonic, antispasmodic, carminative, astringent, alterative

Preparation and Dosage: Using a tincture is recommended because the tea made with this herb is too bitter. It is best to make or purchase the tincture. Tincture dosage is 1" or one dropper full three times a day for chronic conditions. In the case of acute flu symptoms or bronchial distress, you will need to take this more frequently. Take 1" every three to four hours for three days and then gradually reduce as symptoms subside. In acute cases, continue taking the chronic dosage one week after symptoms are gone.

You can make an infusion with one teaspoon of dried root per cup of boiling water. However, the tea is so bitter it may be hard to consume.

Contraindications: Please pay close attention to the botanical characteristics of this plant when harvesting so that you do not confuse it with Snakeroot. Boneset is safe, but Snakeroot is poisonous. The main visual difference is that the Boneset stem is hairy. Look at pictures of these two herbs carefully before you proceed.

Common uses: Boneset was a typical Native American herb used throughout the U.S. for hundreds of years before the settlers arrived. In the 1800s, it was the primary early European settler's treatment for influenza, fevers, liver congestion, and clearing the upper respiratory tract.

Boneset is one of the best remedies for relieving the symptoms of influenza. This herb's pain reduction and expectorant qualities make it a superior herb — it releases chest tightness so bronchioles can drain more quickly. The Native American Indians used it to treat debilitation from fever pains, e.g. breakbone fever or dengue fever. Additionally, it will ease constipation and provide general detoxification.

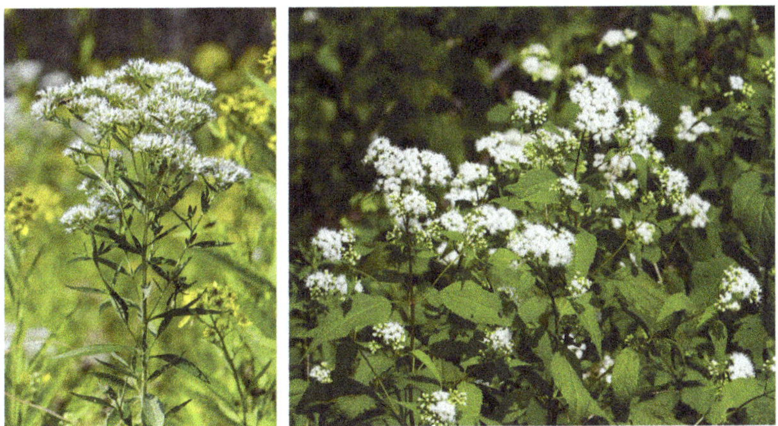

This is Boneset (left) to not confuse with Snakeroot (right)

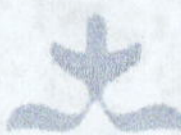

#6 – California Poppy

Eschscholzia Californica, sources: (9) (12)

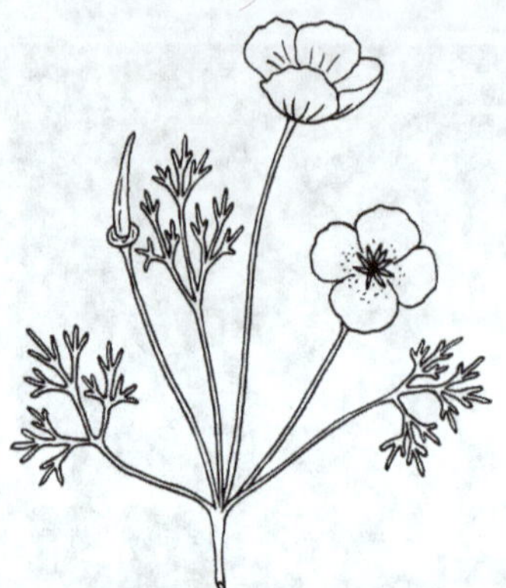

Parts Used: flowers, leaves, seeds

Taste: sweet, to slightly bitter, and astringent

Actions: sedative, nervine, analgesic, antispasmodic, diuretic, anti-inflammatory

Preparation and Dosage: Standard tea dosage applies. Take one teaspoon of the dried flower in one cup of boiling water three times daily.

Contraindications: Please follow the recommended dosage.

Habitat: California poppies grow in open dry, sunny areas, along roadsides, and in gardens across the U.S.

Common uses: The flower soothes anxiety, calms a nervous disposition, and induces a night of sound sleep. California tribes such as the Mendocino and the Costanoan used it as an analgesic. It could also remove lice from hair, and reduce headaches and stomachaches. Poultices of the flower and leaves stop breast milk from flowing when the time comes for weaning a baby. Tribal women in the West applied poppy pollen as eyeshadow.

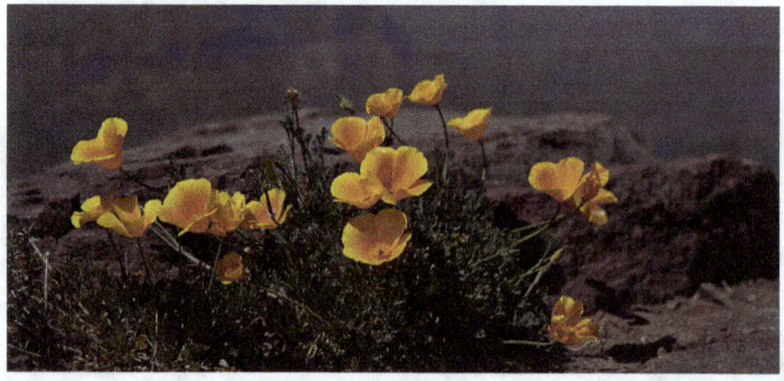

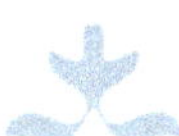

#7 – Cattail

Typha, sources: (10) 11) (18)

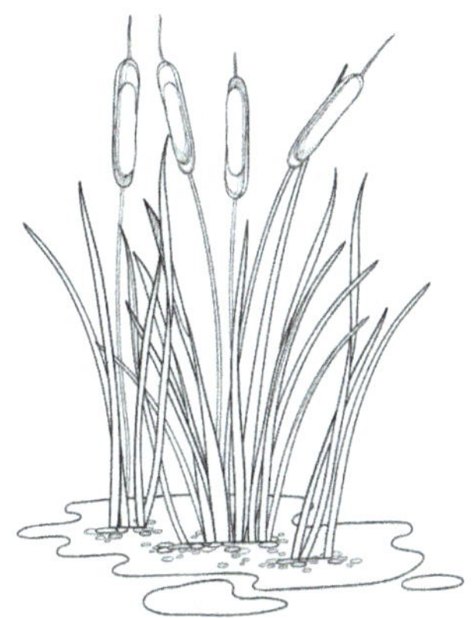

Parts Used: root, seed down, flowers

Taste: sweet to slightly bitter

Actions: anti-bacterial, vulnerary, antidiuretic

Preparation and Dosage: Standard tea dosage applies. Take one teaspoon of the dried root in one cup of boiling water. Boil and mash ½ cup of the root to make a poultice. Wash and chew the flower directly for relief from diarrhea.

Contraindications: Please follow the recommended dosage.

Habitat: Cattails grow in swampy areas with rich soil nationwide, in the sun to part shade.

Common uses: Most tribes who lived near swampy areas used cattails as food and medicine. It was prevalent. Except for the mature leaves and seed heads, all plant parts became medicine. The roots make an effective poultice for healing skin burns and infections. Alternatively, tribe members boiled the starchy roots and mashed them, like mashed potatoes. They ground the seeds into flour for baking and used it for diaper rashes. No part of this plant went to waste. Even the flowers, when eaten directly, stopped diarrhea.

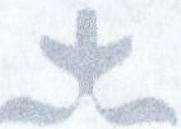

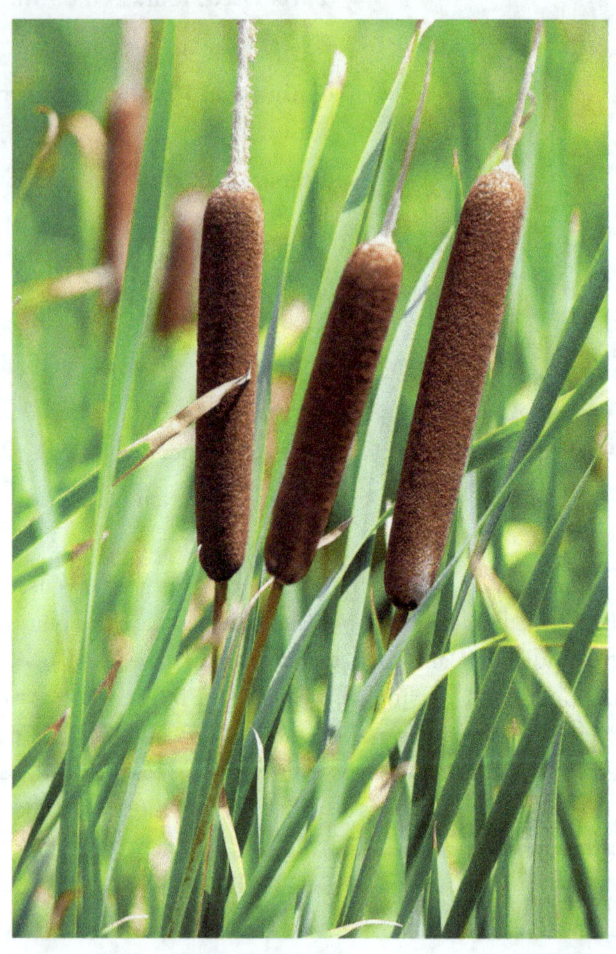

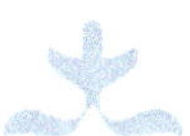

#8 – Chamomile

Matriarcaria Recutita, sources: (3) (6)

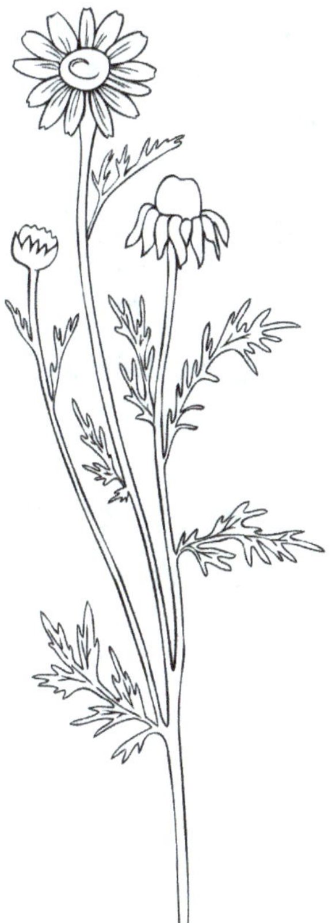

Parts Used: flowering tops

Actions: nervine, adaptogenic, antispasmodic, carminative, anti-inflammatory, antimicrobial, vulnerary

Preparation and dosage: Standard tea dosage applies. Take one teaspoon of the dried flower in one cup of boiling water three times daily.

Contraindications: If you are allergic to ragweed, you will probably be allergic to this plant. Compresses with Chamomile have occasionally produced a rash. In most cases, it is very gentle and safe.

Habitat: German Chamomile is common and does well in poor, clay soil, whereas the Roman variety prefers well-drained and moderately fertile soil. Both types, however, thrive in open, sunny locations. Its cousin, *Pineapple Weed,* grows in gravel and sandy areas (such as driveways). Native American Indians often used Pineapple Weed because it is easier to find than true Chamomile yet has similar medicinal benefits. Pineapple weed is milder.

Common uses: Native American uses of this herb focused on stomach pain, particularly for children. Its benefits are numerous for children and adults. Chamomile alleviates insomnia, anxiety, depression, appetite, menopausal mood swings, diarrhea, aches and pains from flu, migraines, motion sickness, vertigo, conjunctivitis, skin inflammations, and a host of digestive symptoms such as gas, colic pains, or even ulcers.

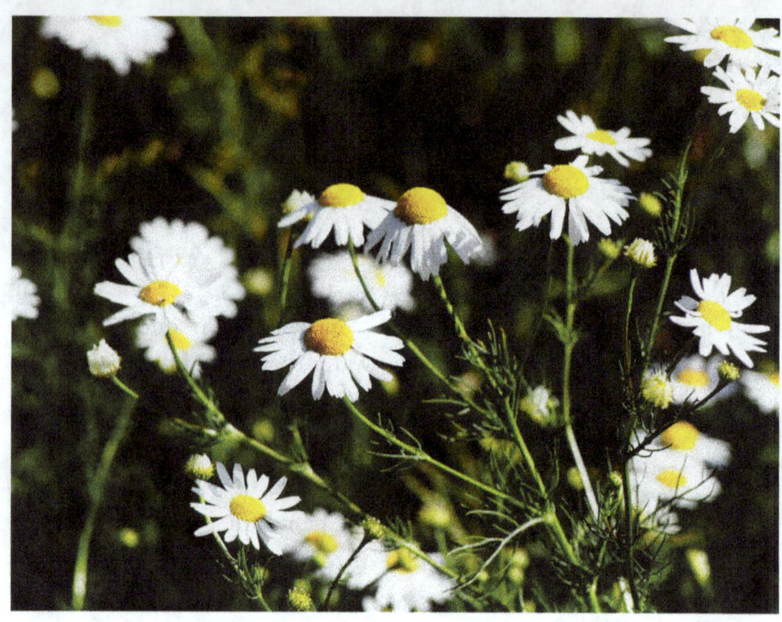

#9 – Dandelion

Taraxacum Officinale, sources: (3) (7) (11)

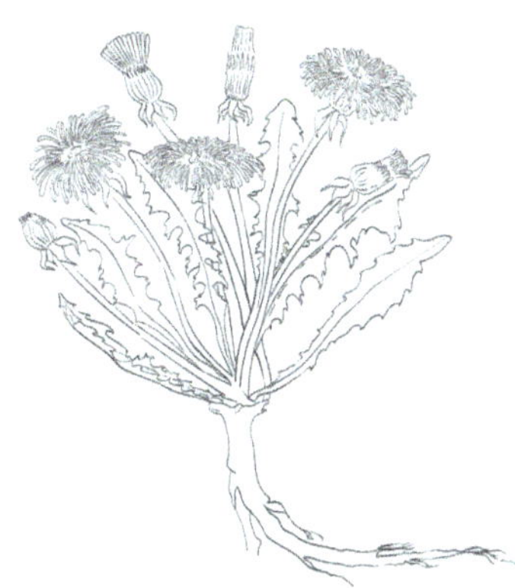

Parts Used: flowers, leaves, roots

Taste: bitter to bittersweet, astringent

Actions: alterative, tonic, diuretic, hepatoprotective, depurative, carminative

Preparation and Dosage: Standard tea dosage applies. Take one teaspoon of the dried flower, leaf or root, in one cup of boiling water three times daily.

Contraindications: Please follow the recommended dosage. Drink plenty of water when consuming this herb to facilitate detoxification.

Habitat: Dandelions thrive on neglect. One finds them in fields, lawns, along forest edges. One sees the swordlike leaves in a rosette formation with small yellow pom flowers attached to the stems.

Common uses: Dandelion is one herb that can cause improvement in almost any condition. Earlier, we have seen how one medicine woman used flowers to remedy mental distress. Native Americans in the Southwest would chop and fry the flowers to make fritters.

Poultices from the roots reach into an infection and reduce it. The leaves stimulate appetite and digestion. They assist with calcium absorption. Dandelion moves blood, so understandably, it benefits liver and gallbladder stagnation. It relieves premenstrual syndrome because it decongests the blood.

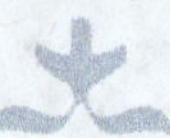

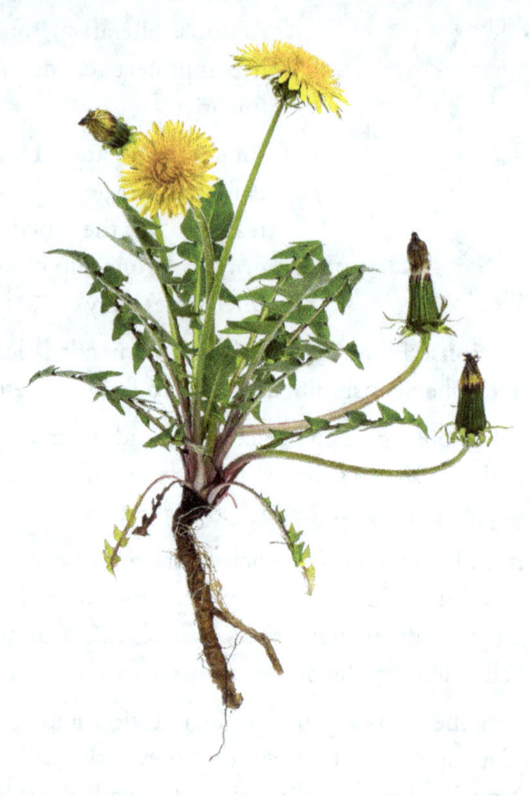

#10 – Devil's Club

Oplopanax Horridus, sources: (16) (17)

Parts Used: rhizomes, roots, stems, and leaves

Actions: antibacterial, adaptogenic, antifungal, and antiviral

Preparation and Dosage:

1. Follow the Standard decoction or a standard tincture dose.

2. Use 1 tablespoon of the fresh root, stem, or leaf per cup of boiling water or one teaspoon of dried herb.

3. Take three cups of tea daily.

Or, take 1" or one dropper full of the tincture three times daily.

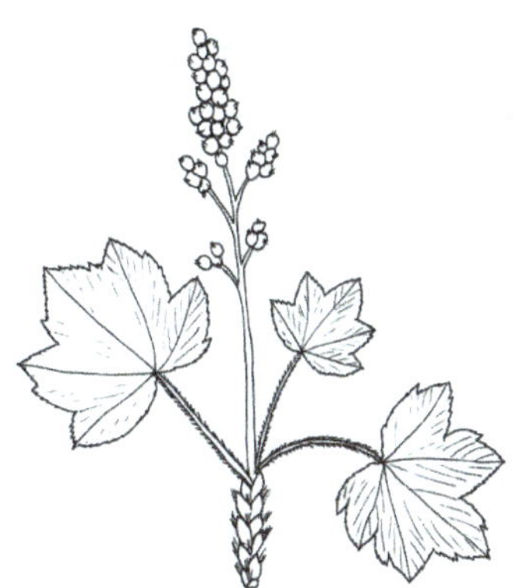

Contraindications: There are no side effects as long as you stay within the recommended dosage range.

Habitat: Devil's Club grows in the undergrowth of mossy coniferous forests, on stony slopes and debris with humid soils. You can find it on river pathways. The stems resemble a very well-developed prickly, wild rose bush.

Common uses: Devil's Club is a famous cousin to American Ginseng. It is known as a potent adaptogen because of its ability to reduce mental and physical fatigue and depression. In Alaska and British Columbia, Native Americans treated arthritis, fever, and diabetes with Devil's Club. Alaskan natives decocted and drank the root to treat cancer by keeping cancer cells from proliferating. Northern Native American tribes in general used, and still use, this herb for arthritis, gallstones, ulcers, constipation, and lingering chest pain, following a cold.

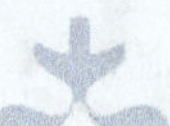

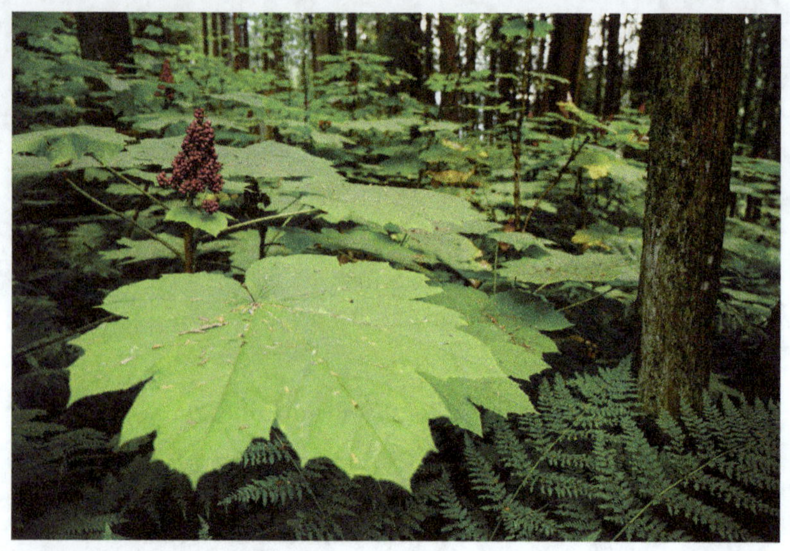

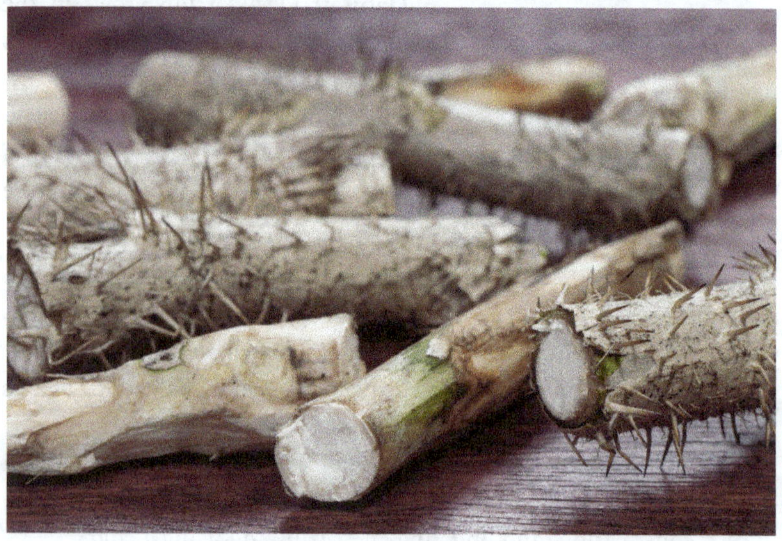

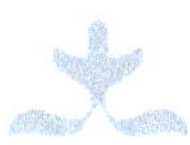

#11 – Echinacea

Echinacea Spp. Compositae, sources: (3) (4) (12) (15)

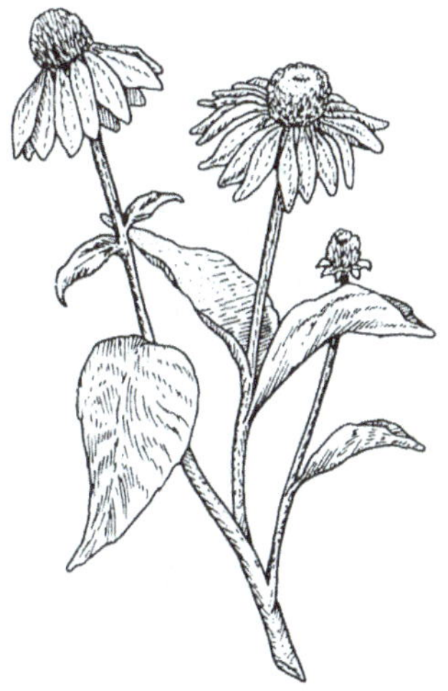

Parts Used: root and aerial portions

Actions: alterative, antibiotic, carminative, stimulant, vulnerary

Preparation and Dosage: Take the Standard Infusion 1 teaspoon of dried leaves and flowers per cup of boiling water. Drink three cups daily. This herb tinctures well and is worth keeping on hand. For chronic, long-term ailments, take 1" of tincture in the morning and evening. For acute conditions like severe inflammation or infections, you will take 1" or one dropper full every three hours until symptoms subside. Then decrease the dosage slowly as you ease into the chronic phase.

Contraindications: Follow the recommended dosage always. This herb is used longer-term, up to six months, very safely.

Habitat: Due to the popularity of this herb, it has been over-harvested, and it is sometimes hard to find. Therefore, it is truly worth cultivating on your own.

Echinacea comes in 9 different species, all of which are native to North America. The visual characteristics of the flower are outstanding. You can see this pink, purplish daisy-like flower from a distance.

Common uses: Echinacea is widely available online due to its popularity. Understandably, the Native Americans used this herb widely. Echinacea alleviates even the most severe inflammatory conditions: boils, skin eruptions, puffy sores, venomous bites, gangrene septicemia, poison oak, and poison ivy. As an antibacterial or antiviral medicine, it is also superior. Within three days of taking the *acute dosage* of Echinacea, acute pus or inflammation should subside, as well as any acute bacterial or viral infections. It is an excellent lymphatic cleanser.

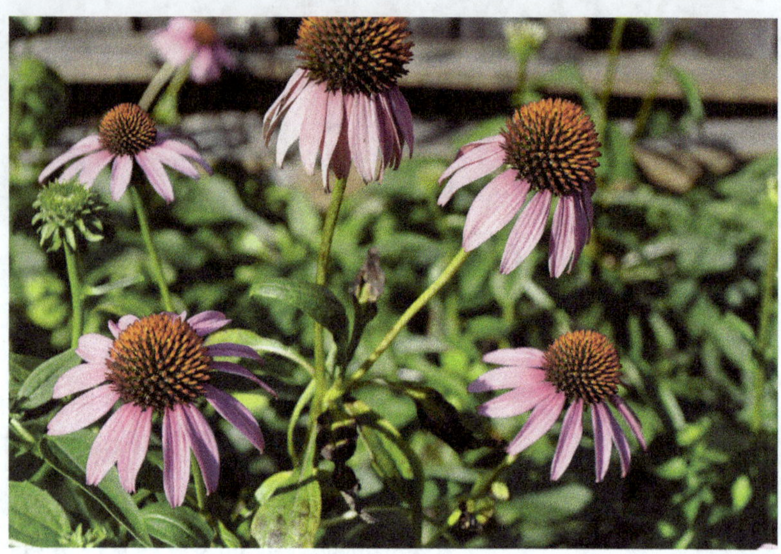

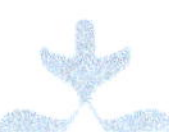

#12 – Elderberry

Sambucus Nigra, sources: (3) (8) (12) (17)

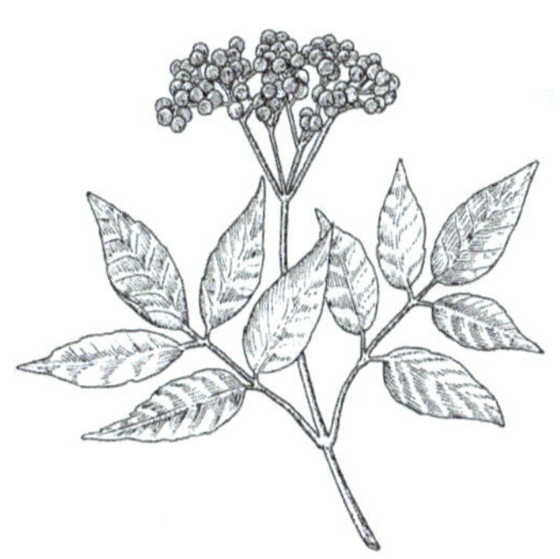

Parts Used: berries, roots, inner bark, leaves.

Taste: sweet, sour, slightly astringent

Actions: antiviral, adaptogenic, anti-inflammatory, cardiotonic, diaphoretic, alterative, emollient

Preparation and Dosage: Standard tea dosage applies. Take one teaspoon of the dried fruit in one cup of boiling water three times daily for ear, nose, and throat issues or flu. Take one teaspoon of the dried root in one cup of boiling water two times daily for constipation. Take one teaspoon of syrup found in the recipe section three times daily in a chronic case of sore throat, cough, or cold. For any critical ailment, such as the flu or bronchitis, take the syrup every three hours.

Contraindications: Please follow the recommended dosage.

Habitat: Elderberry is common throughout plains and mountains in northern and western regions. It is found in wetlands and along streams in the east.

Common uses: Elderberry is a medicine chest must-have for a family. It excels in treating cough, bronchitis, flu, fever, and colds. In general, it reduces inflammation and is an excellent antiviral remedy for children and adults alike. A tea from the bark relieves constipation. The berries help arthritis. It is an ideal herb for children, mainly because they love the taste of syrup. The berries provide strength for adrenal function, as most berries do. Native Americans throughout the North, West, and Eastern regions of the U.S. infused the leaves to treat infections and gave the flowers to colicky children. The berries alleviated rheumatism.

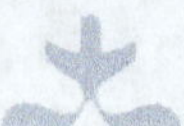

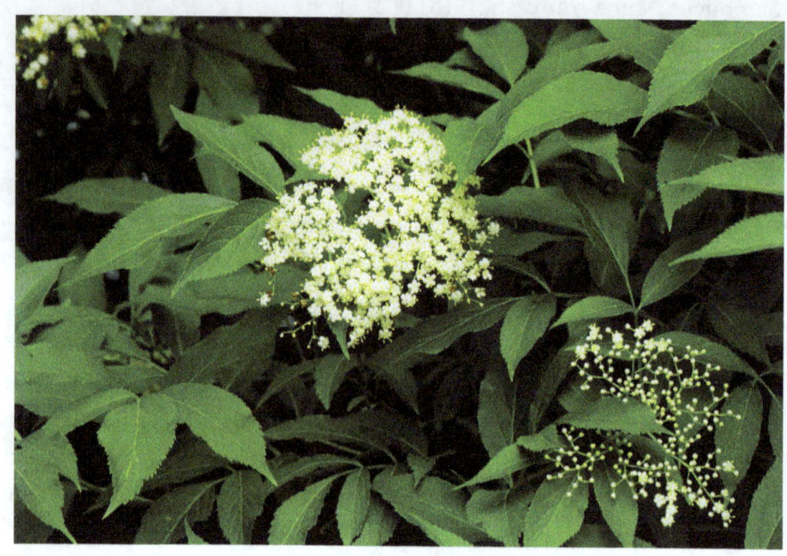

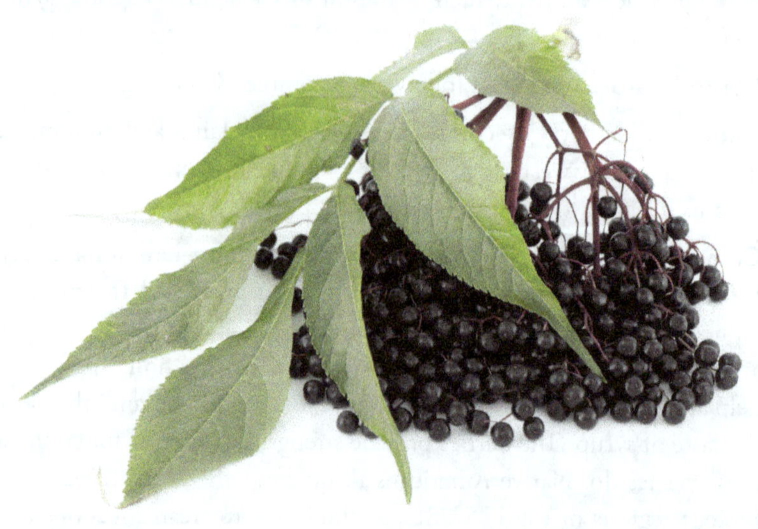

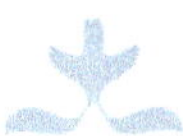

#13 – Ginger

(Asarum Canadense), sources: (6) (12) (13) (17)

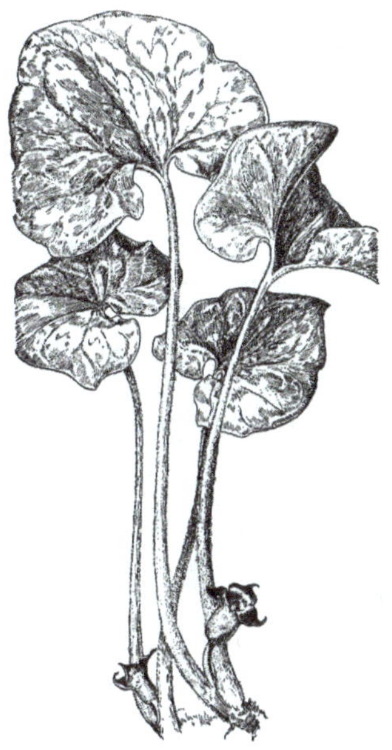

Parts Used: root

Taste: pungent

Actions: stimulant, adaptogenic, carminative, antispasmodic, adaptogenic, rubefacient, diaphoretic, emmenagogue, cardiotonic, hypotensive, expectorant, hypoglycemic, antimicrobial, anti-inflammatory, tonic

Preparation and Dosage: An infusion can be made from one teaspoonful of the fresh root in one cup of boiling water and taken whenever needed as a tonic herb, or at least three times a day for cold, cough, or flu.

Contraindications: Ginger is a tonic and adaptogenic herb that can be used regularly with no contraindications. However, do not take this herb if you suffer from hot flashes. It creates heat.

Habitat: Interestingly, Ginger and Ginseng grow side by side in the wild. You will notice the heart-shaped leaves in the spring in shady low-lying forest beds. Ginseng has curved vein patterns that fan across the leaf side by side. It is an unusual and beautiful design. The root is just below the surface. Harvest, wash, and dry it. If you cannot harvest it yourself, it is one of the most widely applicable and available herbs.

Common uses: The Cherokee Indians used wild Ginger as a carminative, digestive herb, and antiemetic. In Northern forested areas, women boiled a strong decoction from the root as a contraceptive. Ginger relieves morning sickness, chemotherapy-associated nausea, postoperative nausea, and motion sickness. Ginger can potentially treat several ailments, including degenerative disorders such as arthritis and rheu-

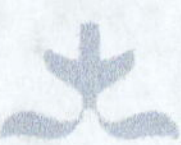

matism, indigestion, constipation and ulcer, and cardiovascular conditions like atherosclerosis and hypertension. On the whole, Ginger contains remarkable anti-inflammatory and anti-oxidative properties for controlling the process of aging.

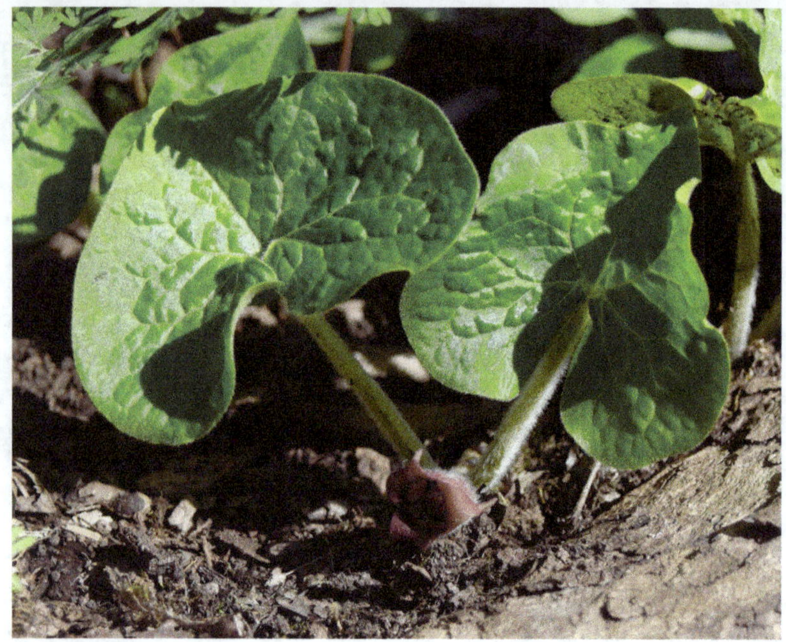

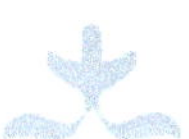

#14 – American Ginseng

Panax Quinquefolius, sources: (6) 12) (17)

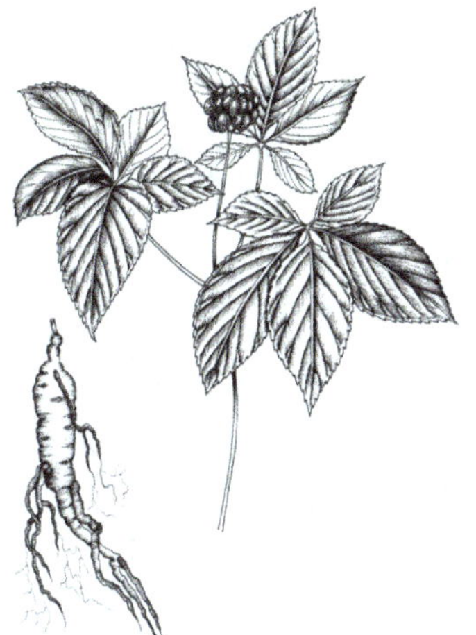

Parts Used: root

Actions: adaptogenic, tonic, stimulant, hypoglycemic

Taste: slightly bitter

Preparation and Dosage: Using the Ginseng root, make a decoction from half a teaspoon of the dried root. It is best to start small with this herb. Take ½ teaspoon in a cup of boiling water three times daily.

Contraindications: Acute inflammatory diseases and bronchitis, headaches, and insomnia. American Ginseng is overly stimulating for these conditions due to its invigorating quality.

Habitat: This is an endangered plant due to overharvesting. If you cannot find it, order it from a sustainable grower. It is still possible to see wild Ginseng on shady forest floors, near ferns, or its cousin wild Ginger. It grows in a specific soil type that contains high calcium.

You will not harvest the plants with two prongs. Wild American Ginseng is endangered. Harvesting the two-pronged plants is illegal. Try to find three-year or preferably five-year growth.

Common uses: Ginseng has an ancient history. It is a powerful adaptogen with a wide range of possible therapeutic uses; it has a tremendous therapeutic application for the weak, the lethargic, and the elderly. Tribes near northern forested areas would use Ginseng as a stimulant for strength on long treks. It was a sexual tonic and aided various conditions like headaches, digestive distress, and female infertility.

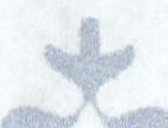

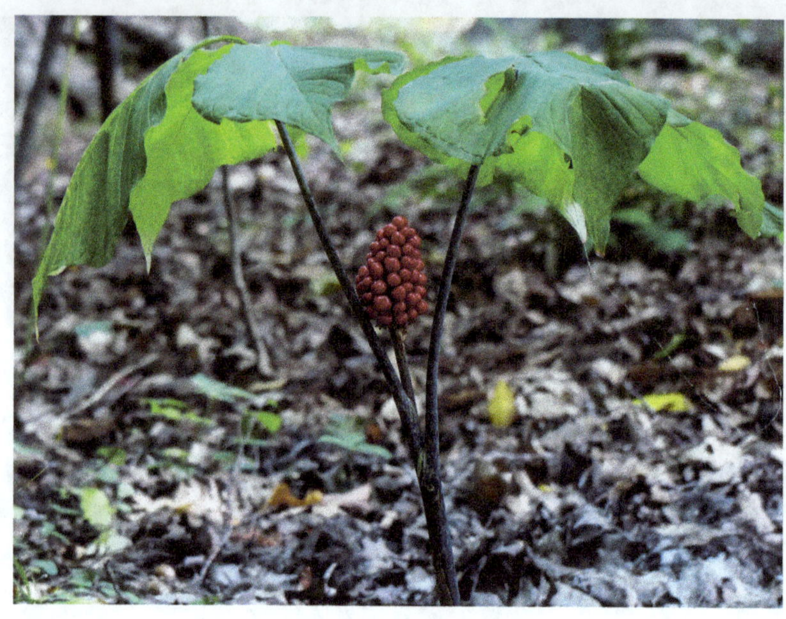

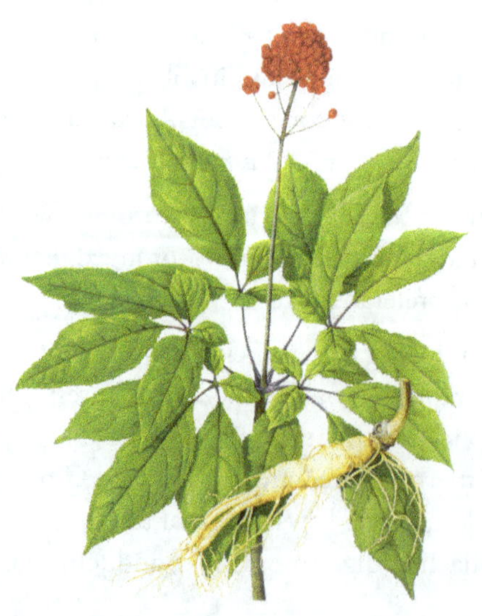

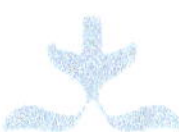

#15 – Goldenrod

Solidago, sources: (3) (11)

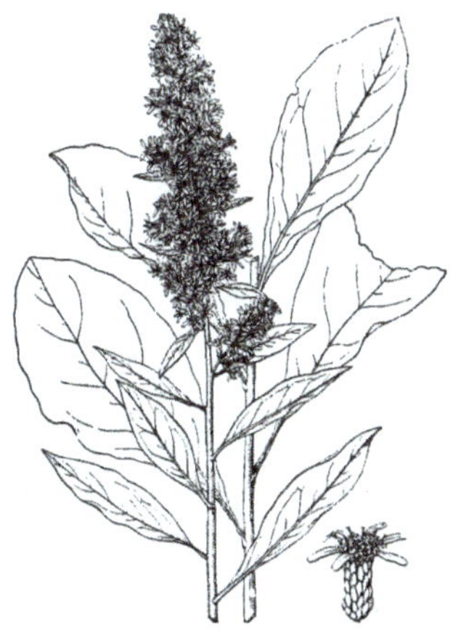

Parts Used: aerial parts

Taste: Slightly bitter, aromatic, slightly sweet

Actions: astringent, stimulating, diaphoretic, diuretic, antiseptic, anti-inflammatory, analgesic

Preparation and Dosage: Make a Standard Infusion: 1 teaspoon dried herb (aerial parts) per cup of boiling water. Drink three cups daily.

Contraindications: Do not take this herb if you have heart or kidney failure. It has a strong diuretic quality.

Habitat: There are more than 125 species of Goldenrod, most of them native to North America for hundreds of years. You will find it in the sun to part shade, meadows and fields. Goldenrod seeds proliferate. Notice the term Solidago meaning solid. The medicine made from it reputedly made you solid or healthy again.

Goldenrod is an easy wildflower to find when it blooms in the fall. Its tall, sturdy stalks and dark green sword-shaped flat leaves have long sprays of small bright gold and yellow flowers on top.

Common uses: Southern, southeastern, and southwestern tribes used Goldenrod extensively. Goldenrod uses vary from relieving influenza, calming repeated colds, soothing bronchitis, or treating tonsillitis, sinusitis, and allergies. It is mainly a respiratory herb. Ironically, many people suffer from Goldenrod allergies. However, being introduced to a tablespoon at a time of the tea over the summer months, while the plant is blooming can sometimes alleviate seasonal Fall allergies.

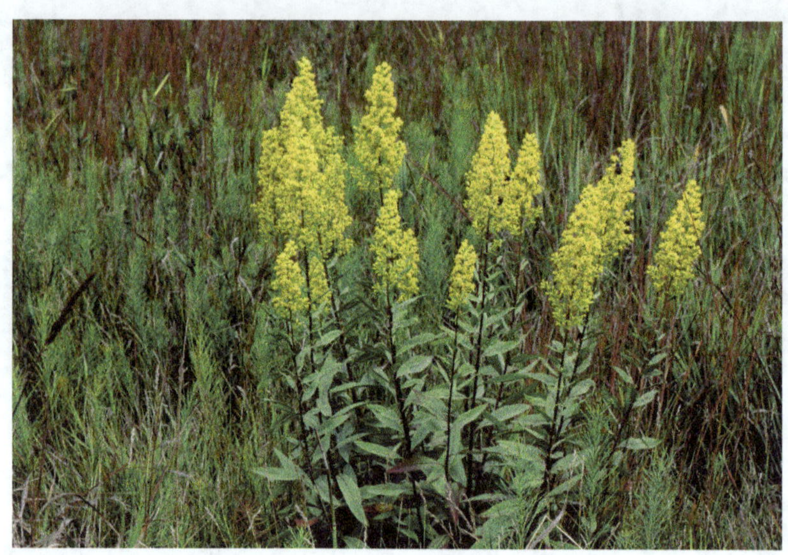

#16 – Green Brier (Sarsaparilla)

Similax Rotundifolia, sources: (6) (22)

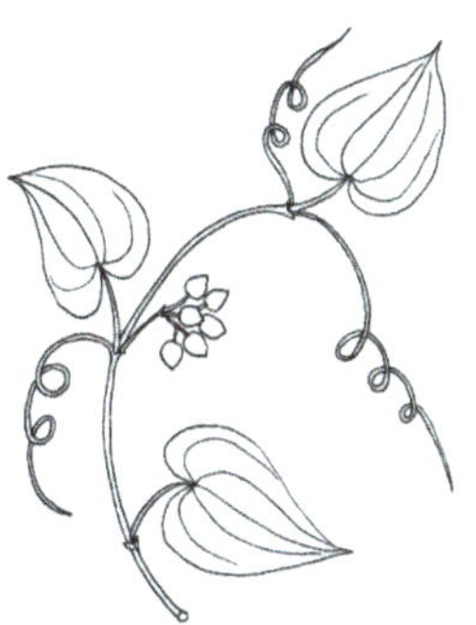

Parts Used: leaves, especially the shoots at the very end of the vines, roots.

Taste: leaves are sour and slightly astringent, the root is sweet and mildly spicy

Actions: astringent, alterative, diuretic, emetic, tonic (leaves contain protein)

Preparation and Dosage:

1. When foraging, gather the leaves. Eat five or six leaves as a natural source of plant protein.

2. Harvest the roots and make a Standard tincture using the simpling method[2]. Take 1" (2.5 cm) or one dropper full three times daily.

3. Dry the roots and make tea with one teaspoon of the dried root in a cup of boiling water. Drink three cups daily.

Contraindications: Greenbrier (Sarsaparilla) has very tangled vines with sharp thorns. Please wear gloves when you are out foraging in general, but especially when you forage this plant!

Habitat: Greenbrier grows low, so low that you might get tangled in it and fall prey to its thorns. It has heart shaped leaves that grow on vines that wrap around trees and other plants in shady forest areas. Notice the vines and the heart-shaped leaves divided by four or five prominent veins. Greenbrier is 20% protein.

---

2   simpling method: Basic method of herbal preparation using a substance to extract the herbs' power.

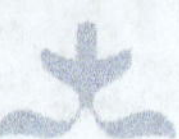

Common uses: This plant is remarkable. Tribes that dwelled in Northern regions used the high protein leaf from Greenbrier as sustenance, particularly while traveling. The Choctaw and Cherokee tribes used the root of this plant, known as Sarsaparilla, to treat skin disorders, liver problems, rheumatism, and excess hormones. However, this herb has ancient uses documented throughout the world.

This herb is an excellent hepatic or liver healer. It is a perfect companion herb to others that heal the blood, such as Yellow Dock, Red Clover, and Dandelion. This herb controls itching.

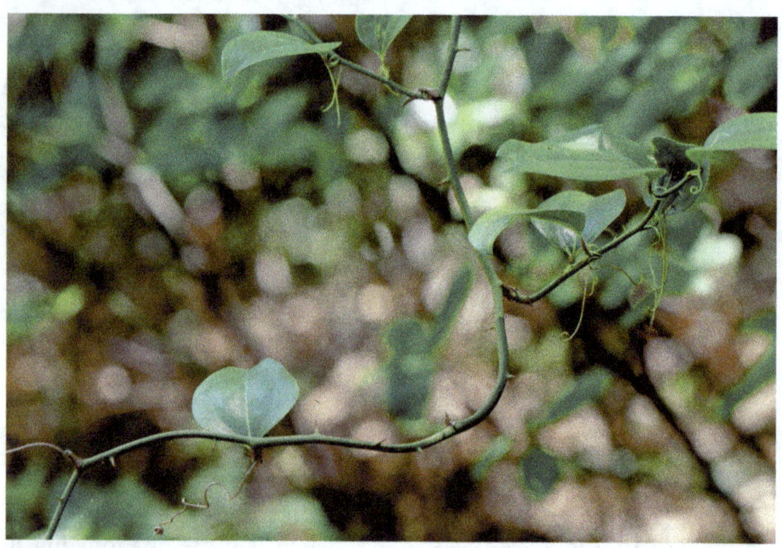

#17 – Hops

Humulus Lupulus, Moraceae, sources: (3)

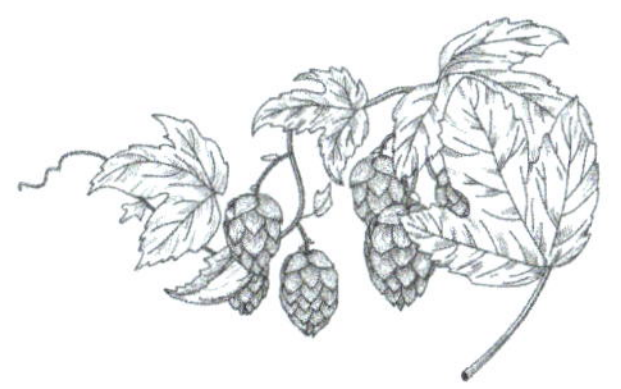

Edible Part Used: flowers, strobiles

Actions: nervine, sedative

Taste: bitter

Preparation and Dosage: Make a Standard Infusion with the flowers one heaping teaspoon per one cup of boiling water. This herb is best used fresh. Take three cups daily.

Contraindications: This is a relatively mild herb.

Common uses: Relieves insomnia, nervous tension, anxiety, restlessness, headache restlessness, indigestion, and mucus in the stool. Across the North, various tribes discovered Hops as a sedative and sleep aid. Also, it relieves toothaches and digestive issues. Don't forget that Hops are one constituent of beer.

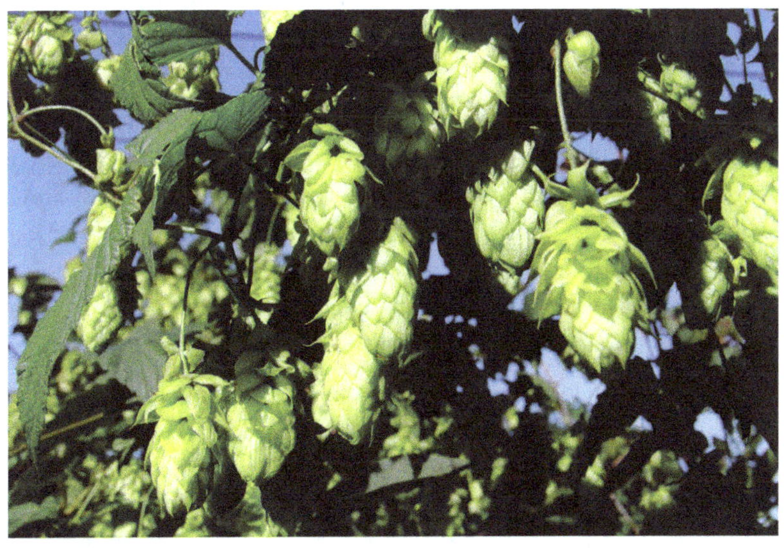

#18 – Horsetail

Equisetum Arvense, sources: (3) (12) (23)

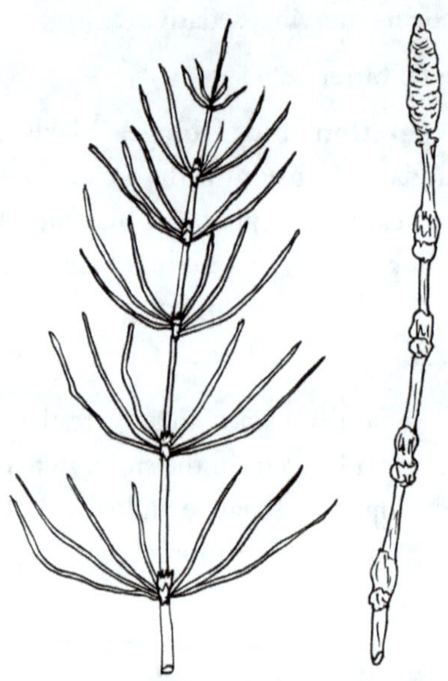

Parts Used: dried aerial stems

Taste: astringent, neutral to slightly bitter

Actions: astringent, diuretic, tonic, vulnerary

Preparation and dosage: Make a tea using one teaspoon of the dried stems per cup of boiling water. Take this three times daily. This herb does not tincture very well.

Contraindications: Please follow the recommended dosage. There is a slight possibility of ingesting toxins if you overdose in large quantities. It is better to use this herb under the guidance of a practitioner.

Habitat: Horsetail grows in rocky or sandy, well-drained soil, often along the road's edge in forested areas. It can also grow in more swampy conditions. It is an unmistakable herb that dates back to the Paleozoic Era. The sturdy stalks extend upwards with large needle-like projections fanning out from around the circumference of the stem. Early settlers used this plant to scrub pots and pans!

Common uses: Horsetail is a common Blackfoot, Cherokee, and Northwestern tribal herb. It is a mild diuretic. It tones and acts as an astringent for the genito-urinary system. It makes a good poultice because it contains silica, an essential mineral that strengthens all connective tissues and heals the skin. Horsetail fortifies the kidneys. It works for incontinence and bedwetting with children.

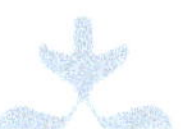

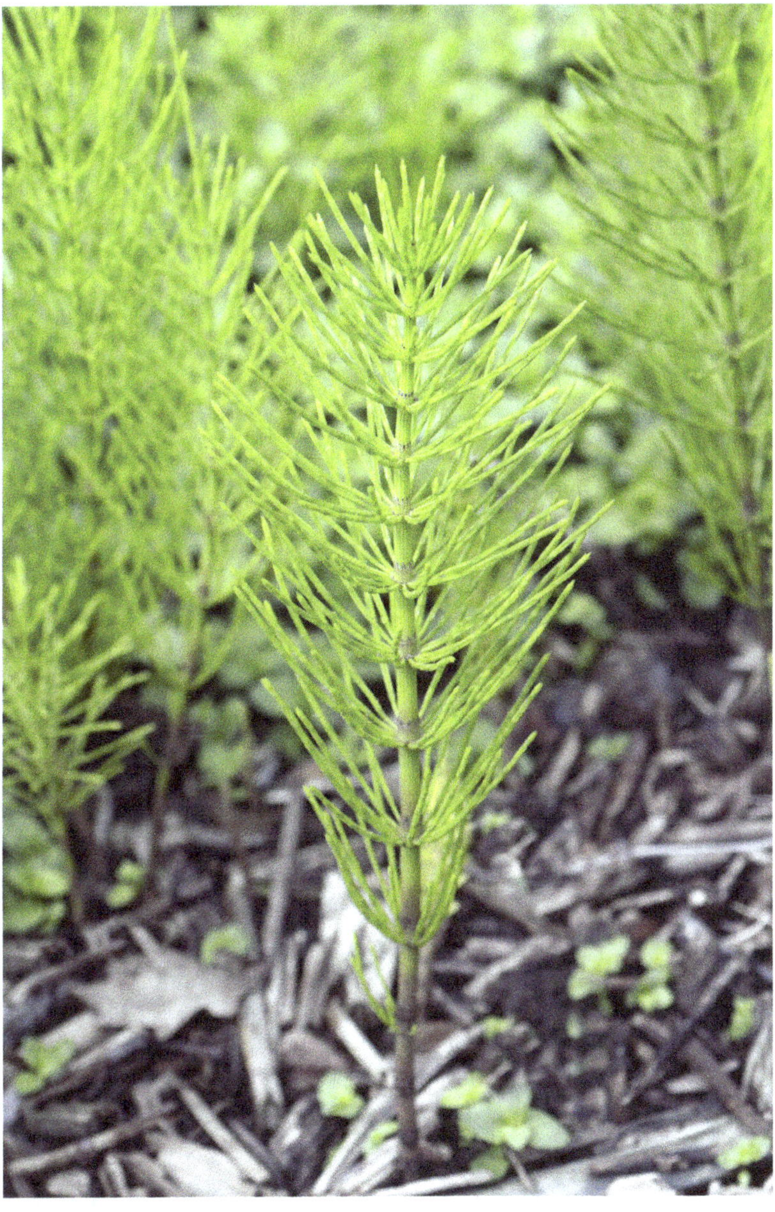

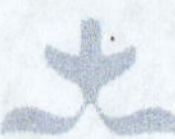

#19 – Lemon Balm

Melissa Officinalis, sources: (3) (6) (10) (12) (17)

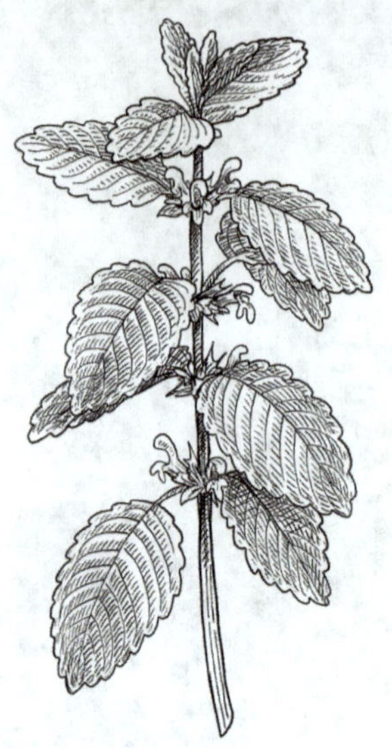

Parts Used: aerial parts

Taste: aromatic

Actions: carminative, nervine, adaptogenic, antispasmodic, antidepressant, diaphoretic, antimicrobial, hepatic

Preparation and Dosage: Make a Standard Infusion with one teaspoon of the dried herb or in a cup of boiling water. Take three cups daily.

Contraindications: Follow the recommended dosage. It is a very gentle herb. It can easily be used with the elderly and also with children.

Habitat: Lemon Balm has a square stem-like all members of the mint family. It can tolerate various soils and prefers sunny locations at elevations up to approximately 3,200 ft (1000 m). Once found in the wild, Lemon Balm is primarily grown in gardens. Its foliage usually has a mild lemon fragrance; otherwise, this plant is similar to several other species in the Mint family, with small purplish to whitish flowers.

Common uses: Like Chamomile, Lemon Balm is a superior herb for digestive spasms. It helps with anxiety or depression symptoms and effects from tension or neuralgia. It relieves palpitations coming from anxiety or insomnia. It made a perfect ceremonial herb and a medicinal one for tribes throughout the U.S.

This plant interfaces between the digestive tract and nervous system. This is an action of high value because it is a neurorestorative herb and digestive tonic herb, all at once. Lemon Balm works well for headaches. It also aids the heart and circulatory system. As a vasodilator, it will lower blood pressure. When you have the flu, this herb is a great companion as it has excellent antiviral properties. It can alleviate feverish conditions while calming the nerves. Its antimicrobial components are noteworthy. Lemon Balm is one of the best herbs to keep for children.

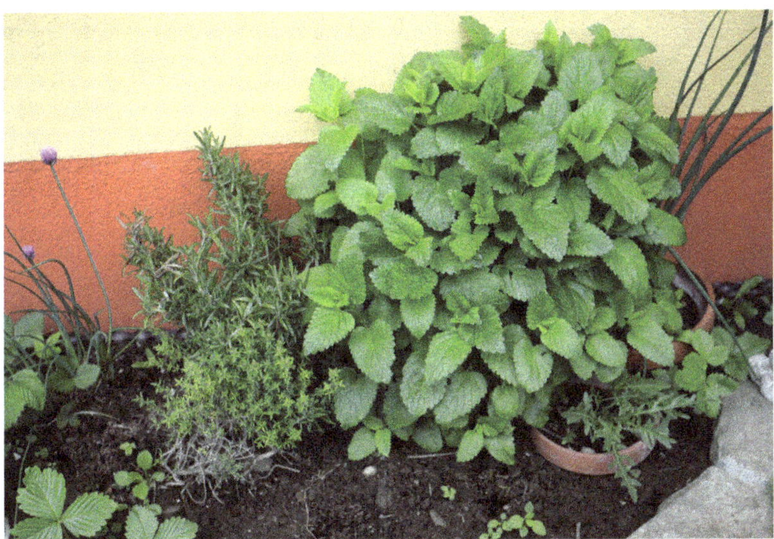

#20 – Milkweed

Asclepias Speciose, sources: (9) (3)

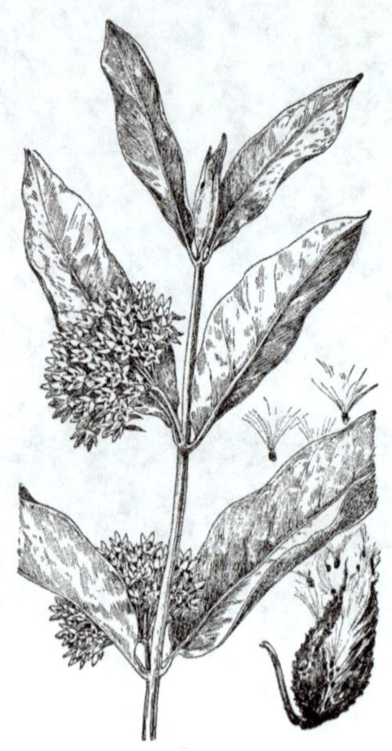

Parts Used: seeds, flowers, roots (leaves used externally only)

Taste: bitter

Actions: cardiotonic, expectorant, anti-tumor, diuretic

Preparation and Dosage: Standard tea dosage applies. Take one teaspoon of the dried flower or root in one cup of boiling water three times daily. Do not use the leaves to make tea. They contain too much oxalic acid.

Contraindications: Please follow the recommended dosage. The leaves can be toxic if consumed internally. Only use them externally.

Habitat: Commonly found in open, sunny meadows and fields. It grows up to 4-6 ft tall (1-2 m) with pink to purple flowers in a cluster.

Common uses: Milkweed is a superior herb for bronchial conditions. It dries up congestion and mucus in the lungs and expels it. Native American tribes used it as a cardiotonic and respiratory tonic through-out the West. It heals gastritis and kidney disorders. Similar to Yellow Dock, it cleanses the blood. The sap heals wounds of all types, even ringworm, and extracts poison from the skin. Western tribes made flour from the seeds and chewed on the root to alleviate sore throats and rashes.

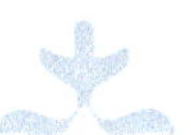

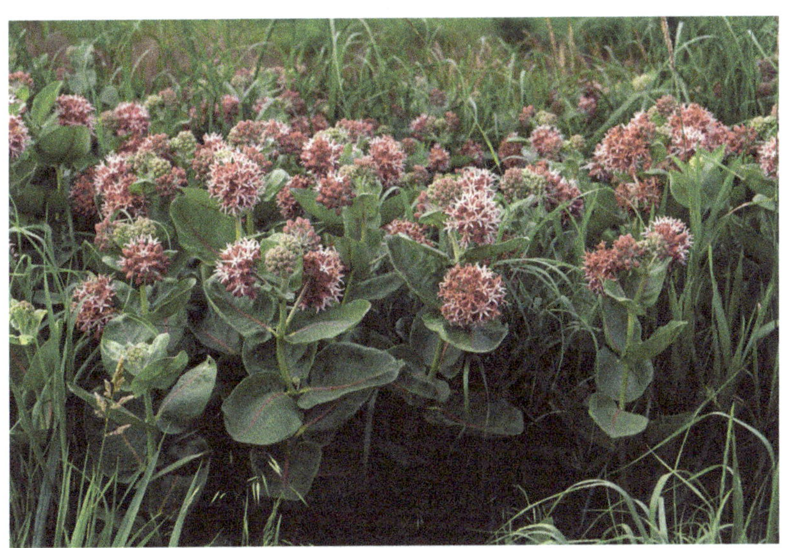

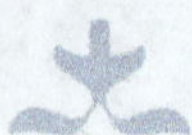

#21 – Meadowsweet

Filipendula Ulmaria, sources: (6) (9) (11)

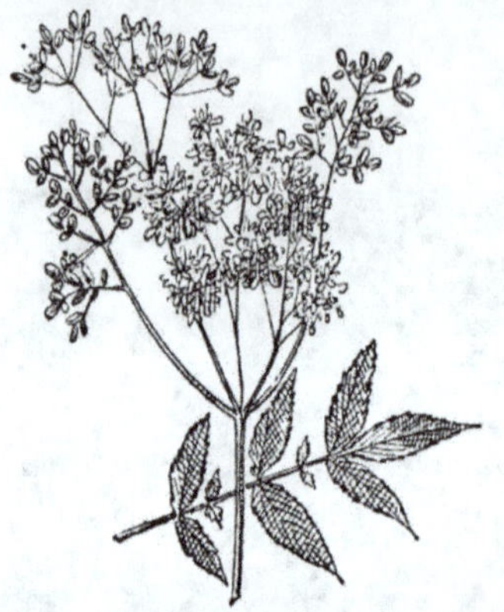

Parts used: aerial parts

Temperature: warming

Taste: bitter

Actions: anti-rheumatic, anti-inflammatory, carminative, antacid, anti-emetic, astringent

Preparation and Dosage: Standard Infusion applies; take one teaspoon of the dried herb in one cup of boiling water. Drink three cups daily.

Contraindications: Please follow the recommended dosage. Meadowsweet is an astringent herb. Drink plenty of water while you take it to rehydrate.

Habitat: Meadowsweet or Mead Wort is a perennial herb that grows in damp meadows. It is native throughout most of Europe and Western Asia. Now it is commonly grown throughout North America. It is a stately-looking plant that can grow up to 5 ft tall (1.5 m). The dark brown stems are thick and crowned with a tip spray of tiny white flowers in a cone shape.

Common uses: North American tribes used Meadowsweet as an excellent digestive remedy that is effective for protecting and soothing the mucous membranes of the digestive tract. Native Americans introduced this herb to settlers. It reduces acidity and eases nausea; therefore, it is very calming in the treatment of heartburn. Its astringent quality helps decrease diarrhea. Meadowsweet does contain salicylic acid (the same substance used in aspirin) not as much as in White Willow, but it still can reduce inflammation. It relieves fever, rheumatism, arthritis, and other joint aches.

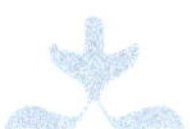

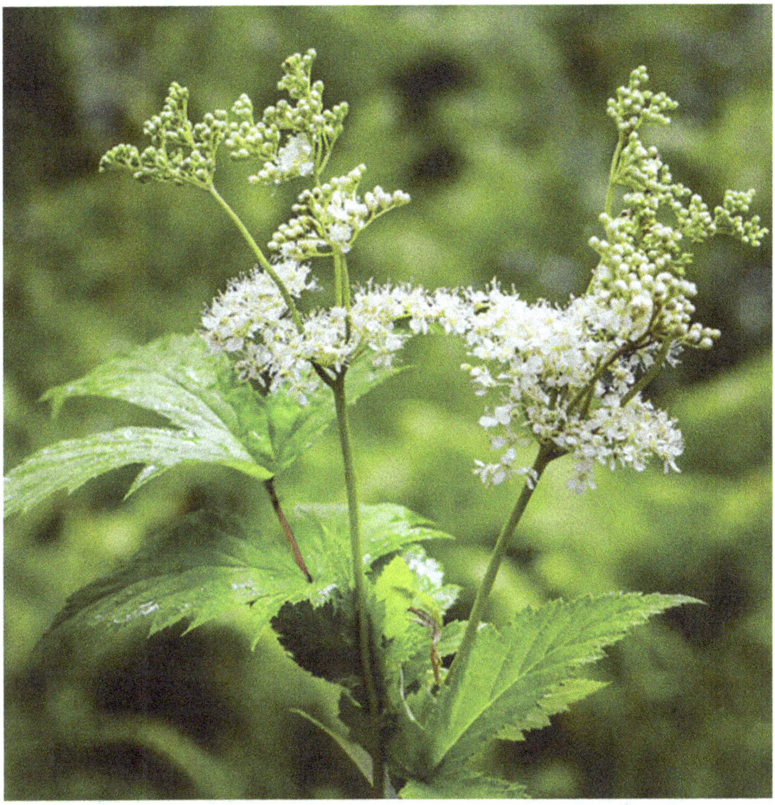

#22 – Mint

Mentha Piperita, sources: (2) (3) (6)

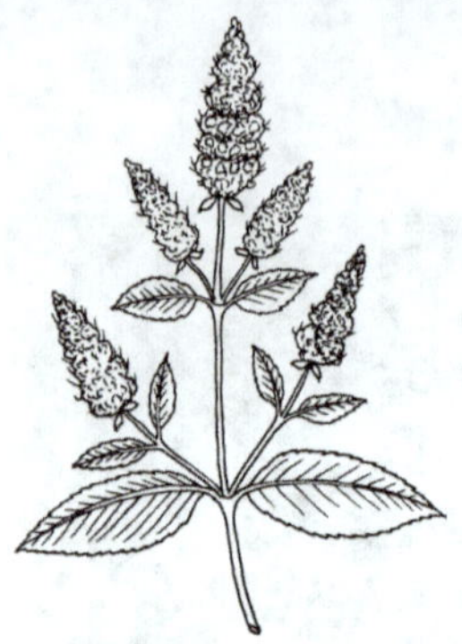

Parts used: aerial parts

Taste: aromatic, slightly bitter

Actions: nervine, antimicrobial, analgesic, aromatic, antispasmodic, anti-inflammatory, carminative, diaphoretic, antiemetic, biliary

Preparation and Dosage: Make a Standard Infusion with one teaspoon of the dried herb per cup of boiling water. Drink three cups daily.

Contraindications: Mint is safe. Follow the recommended dosage.

Habitat: Wild Mint is a common Mint family plant of moist meadows and moist areas around marshes and streams. It grows from rhizomes and spreads by rhizome growth, forming colonies. Full sun is preferred, but partial shade is tolerated.

Common uses: Wild Mint will have most of the same benefits as Peppermint. This profile focuses on Peppermint. First of all, it is a wonderful carminative; it relaxes the spasms in the digestive system's muscles; it can also assist with flatulence. It relieves intestinal colic, dyspepsia, and similar conditions. Peppermint or any Mint can ease nausea during pregnancy or travel sickness. Peppermint can treat ulcerations in the bowels.

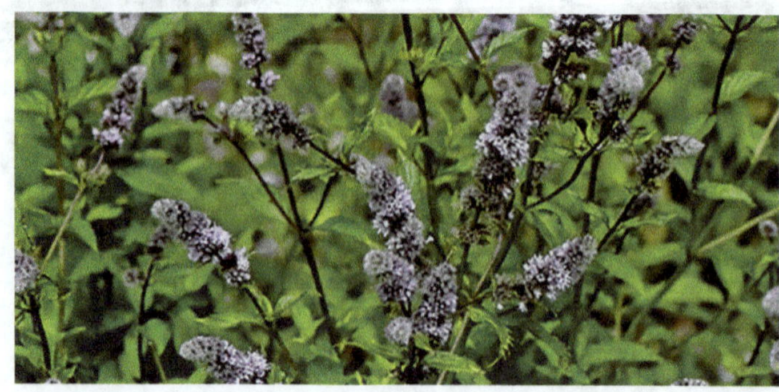

#23 – Mugwort

Artemisia Vulgaris, sources: (3) (8)

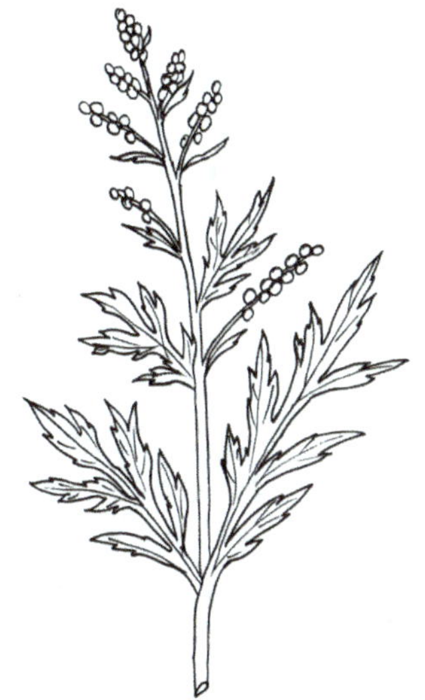

Parts used: leaves

Taste: bitter, acrid

Actions: vermifuge, emmenagogue, hemostatic, antispasmodic, diaphoretic, mild narcotic, bitter tonic

Preparation and Dosage: Make a Standard Infusion with one teaspoon of the dried herb in 1 cup of boiling water. Take 3 cups daily.

Contraindications: Avoid using during pregnancy.

Habitat: *Artemisia vulgaris* proliferates in high-elevation pastures, forest edges, valleys, hillside wastelands, ditches, and roadsides. The stems are branched and purplish brown. The ascending stems have short hairs. The lobed leaf version is widespread in the Northeast. It has medium-sized lobed leaves that are dark green on the top and papery white underneath.

Common uses: Mugwort treats the liver, stomach, and intestinal problems. It is an excellent remedy for worms. It is also a noteworthy herb for controlling shaking induced by nervousness or insomnia. The tincture treats liver and stomach disorders. Mugwort is an *extremely bitter* herb. Native Americans used it for colds, flu, bronchitis, fevers, and ceremonial purposes.

Bundles of it are rolled and lit like incense throughout Asia. It has a musky, earthy smell when it is burned and is somewhat sedative. When Native Americans migrated to the Americas, they brought this practice. Mugwort is applied topically in a poultice or taken as tea internally to stop hemorrhaging or bleeding.

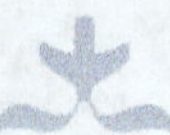

Poultices from the leaves serve to heal wounds. The Dakota, Cheyenne, and Blackfoot tribes used the fresh root to treat rheumatism. The Iroquis mashed the root and applied it to soothe hemorrhoids.

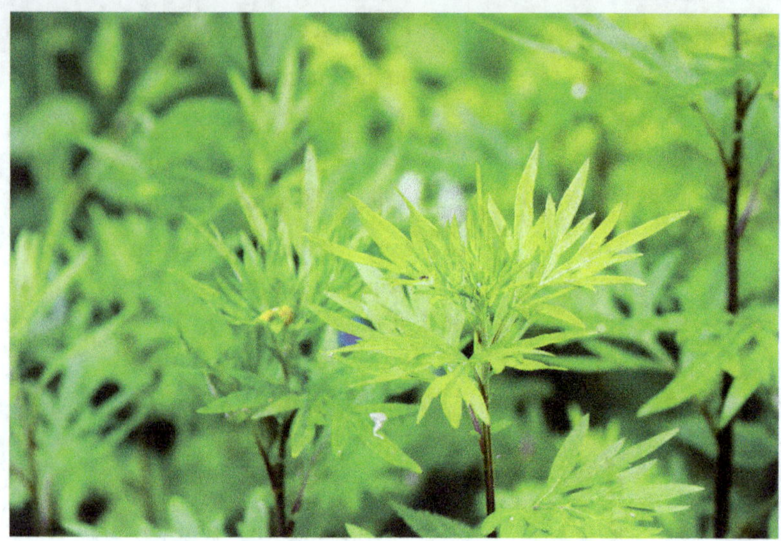

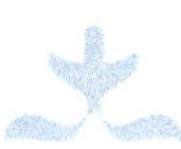

#24 – Mullein

Verbascum Thapsus, sources: (3) (9) (12)

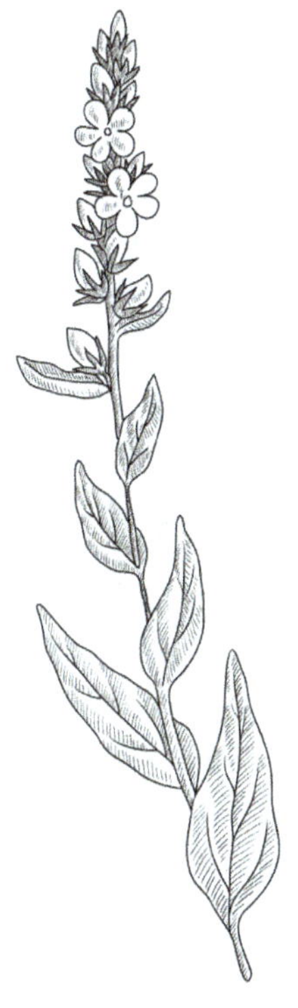

Parts used: leaf flower and root

Taste: slightly bitter

Actions: expectorant, demulcent, antispasmodic, antitussive, astringent, and vulnerary

Preparation and Dosage: Make a Standard Infusion with one teaspoon of the dried leaves or flowers in 1 cup of boiling water. Take three cups daily.

Contraindications: Please follow the recommended dosage.

Habitat: Mullein is a striking plant. It is a biennial that comes from Europe. It thrives in turbid waste areas in part shade to part sun. However, it grows in full sun in waste areas or barren areas. It sends an impressive yellow floral spike up through a silvery green base of leaves. This plant grows on roadsides, sunlit gravel, or sandy areas.

Common uses: You could call this herb the ideal family herb. Mullein is for bronchial and lung congestion; it is a gentle enough herb for children and the elderly. Often, it can ease lymphatic congestion. It is effective in dry, irritated bronchial tissues resulting from a consistent dry hacking cough, a respiratory infection, or smoking. It was a traditional remedy for tuberculosis and could calm the coughing spasms of the lungs.

The leaves are so sturdy and soft that they are called "nature's toilet paper." Native American mothers would use them just like a baby diaper. The plant compounds healed diaper rash directly. Native Americans sometimes made necklaces from the dried root for teething children to reduce pain.

Mullein ear oil, found in the recipe section, is effective for throbbing in the ear or pain from an ear infection. The antimicrobial, anti-inflammatory actions not only heal ear infections but soothe the outside of a jaw with TMJ if one applies the oil externally and lays a hot water compress over it.

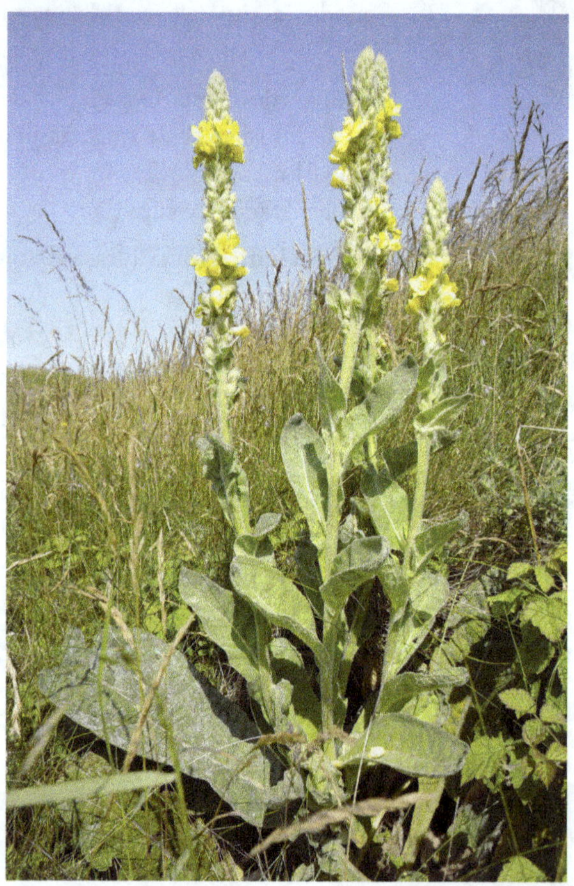

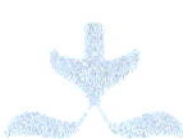

#25 – Mushrooms

Fungi: sources: (17)

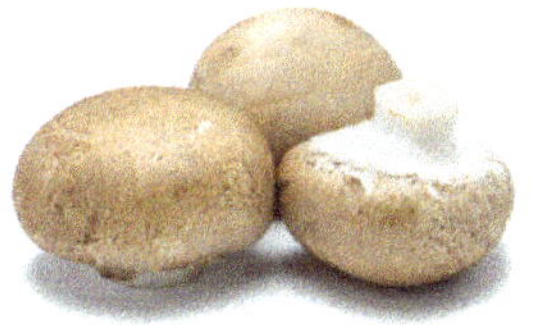

Parts Used: stem and cap

Taste: sweet, woody

Actions: tonic, adaptogenic, enhances cognition, and increases longevity

Preparation and Dosage: Take one teaspoon of the dried mushroom three times daily with food.

Contraindications: Common white button mushrooms, crimini, portobello, Reishi, and Maitake mushrooms are in grocery stores. Outside of these varieties, foraging mushrooms requires skill. Many mushrooms are highly poisonous. ***Please review this link to classes on mushroom identification. This book only provides a brief introduction to this critical plant species.***[3]

Habitat: Many common edible mushrooms feed off the decay of trees. So, learn to identify these trees and how to avoid poisonous mushrooms first. Decaying oak trees, maple trees, willow trees, and alder trees produce colonies of mycelium that become pins or baby mushrooms and then fully mature after a week to two weeks. It is worth repeating — learn to identify your trees first, then learn to identify safe mushrooms for consumption. It cannot be overemphasized.

Common uses: Native American Indians did not only harvest mushrooms for ceremonial, trance-inducing states. They also understood the potency of fungi medicinally. More research is needed before we know all of the various ways Native American tribes utilized mushrooms as medicine. For instance, they harvested Fomitopsis officinalis, generated from the decay of conifer trees.

---

3   Adam Haritan, a botanist provides a wealth of knowledge about how to forage mushrooms safely. *Introduction To Wild Mushrooms with Adam Haritan (Learn Your Land) — YouTube*

Particularly during pandemic times, research on fungi abounds. Science has demonstrated its capacity to stabilize mood, enhance cognitive abilities and increase longevity. Traditional Chinese medicine has reported these benefits for thousands of years.

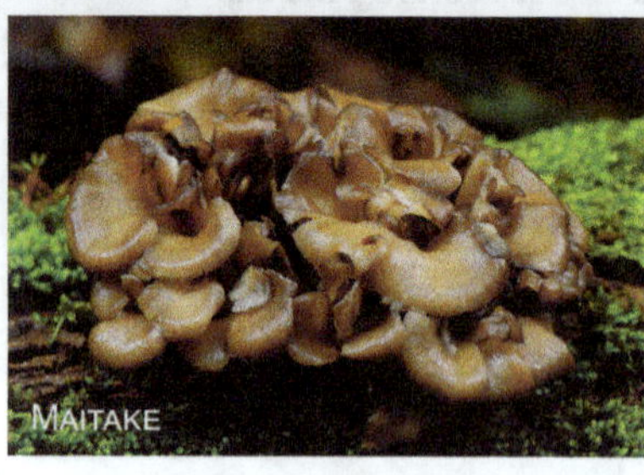

MAITAKE

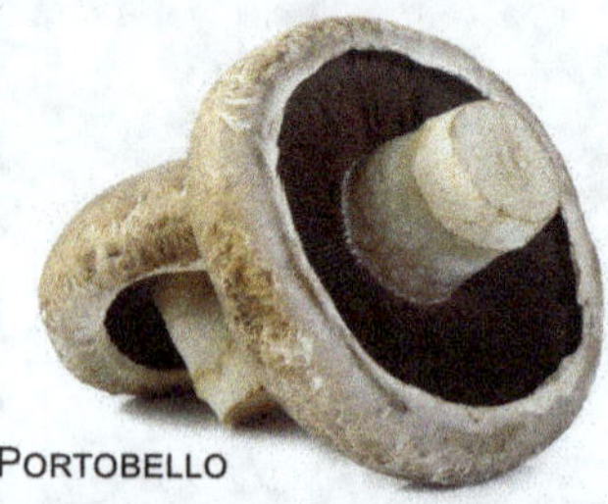

PORTOBELLO

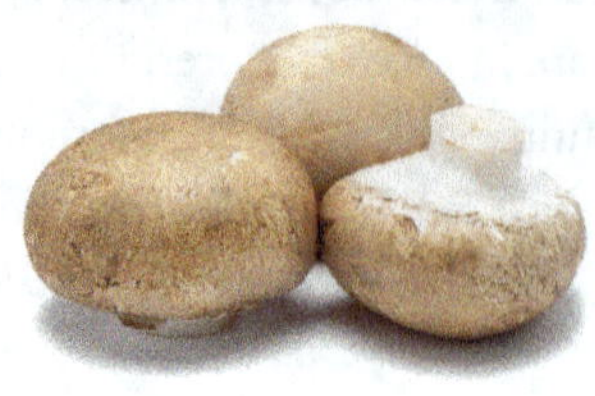

CRIMINI

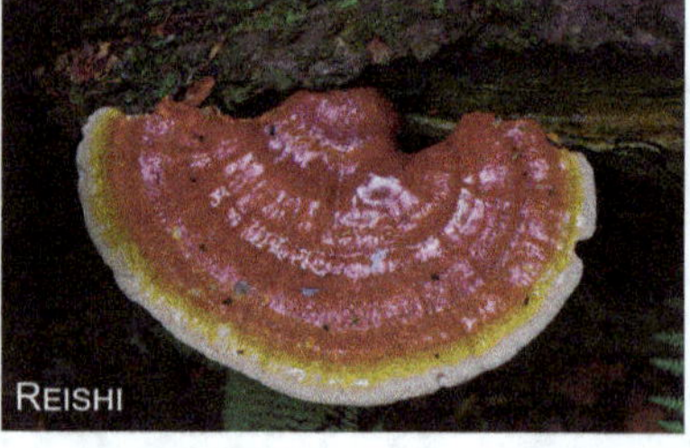

REISHI

#26 – Nettle

Urtica Dioica, sources: (6) (9) (12) (17)

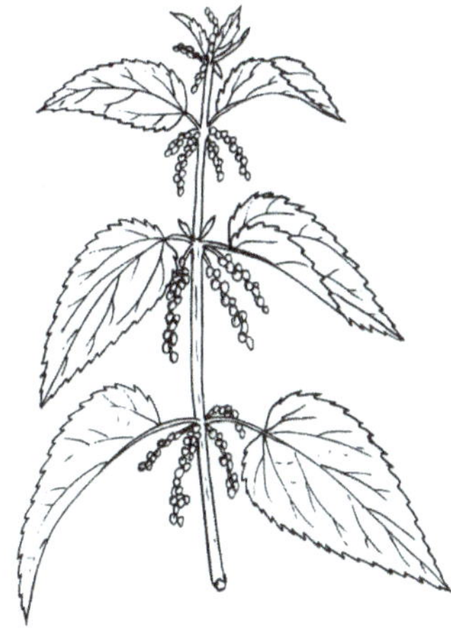

Parts Used: leaves

Taste: bitter

Actions: detoxification, tonic, antihistamine, immunostimulating, adaptogenic, expectorant

Preparation and Dosage: Standard tea dosage applies. Take one teaspoon of the dried leaf in one cup of boiling water three times daily. Or, if you have access to the fresh leaves, cook them like spinach and take 2 oz to 4 oz a few times a week.

Contraindications: Please follow the recommended dosage. Nettles are a strong detoxifying herb. Detoxifying too quickly or without drinking enough water may cause a headache.

Habitat: Nettles thrive in the sun to part shade. They prefer damp, wooded areas with rich soil. You may find them by rivers and streams. Please note that a close cousin to Nettle is Blessed Thistle, also widely used by native tribes in all regions of the U.S.

Common uses: Nettles are both a superfood and a full-spectrum herb. They are incredibly high in minerals, calcium, magnesium, potassium, iron, phosphorus, manganese, and silica. They are an excellent source of vitamin C, B vitamins, and chlorophyll. Nettles are perfect for immune support and reduce most allergic responses. They restore kidney and liver function, build blood and alleviate anemia. If a person is weak from illness or chronically sick from any ailment, Nettle is a great recovery herb.

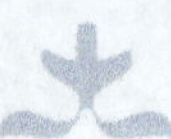

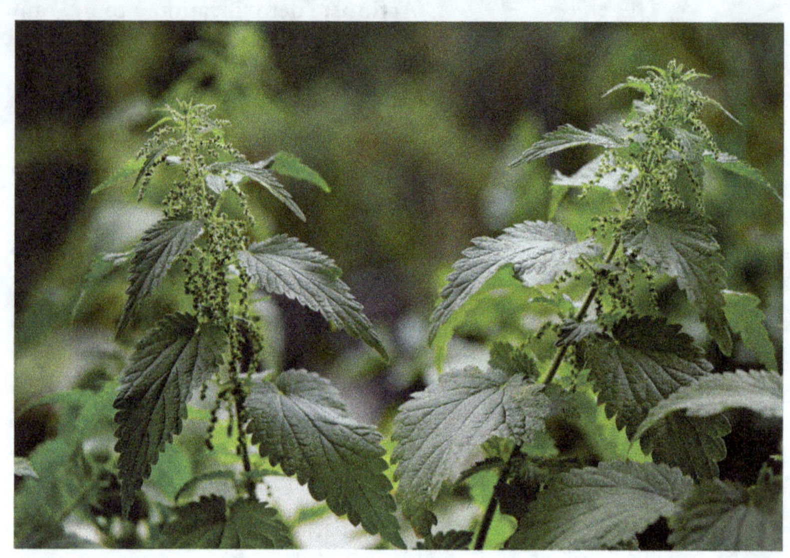

#27 – Oak

Quercus, spp., Faceae, sources: (8) (24)

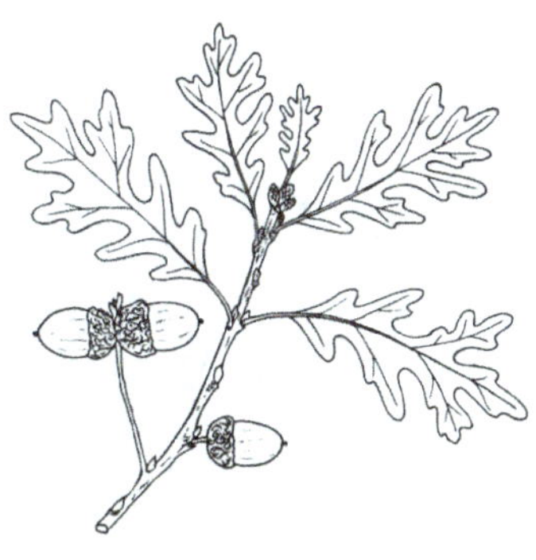

Parts Used: leaves, oak galls, roots, bark fruit (acorns)

Taste: astringent, slightly bitter

Actions: Astringent, antiseptic, anti-diarrheal (one could say acorns have an adaptogenic quality)

Preparation and Dosage: Standard tea dosage applies. Take one teaspoon of the dried bark or root in one cup of boiling water three times daily.

Contraindications: Please follow the recommended dosage.

Habitat: Over ninety species of Oak grow in the U.S. Leaves are lobed, round, or pointed depending on the species. This tree is easy to spot and generally has acorns on it or on the ground beneath it. Acorns can take six to 18 months to mature!

Common uses: A decoction of the bark or root is used as a mouthwash to reduce canker sores or drunk as a tea to reduce muscle and joint pain or inflammation. Oak bark tea relieves dysentery and edema. It is a bronchial remedy as well. Native Americans commonly applied acorn flour as a poultice on sores or other skin conditions to extract toxins. Acorns contain the full medicinal benefits of this tree. Interestingly, many Native American tribes knew that acorn mush is one of the best foods to help a weak and debilitated body following an illness. Native American elder Dennis Martinez, tells how his ancestors, from the O'odham and Chicano heritage called the Oak "the tree of life".

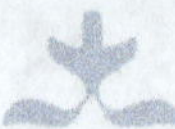

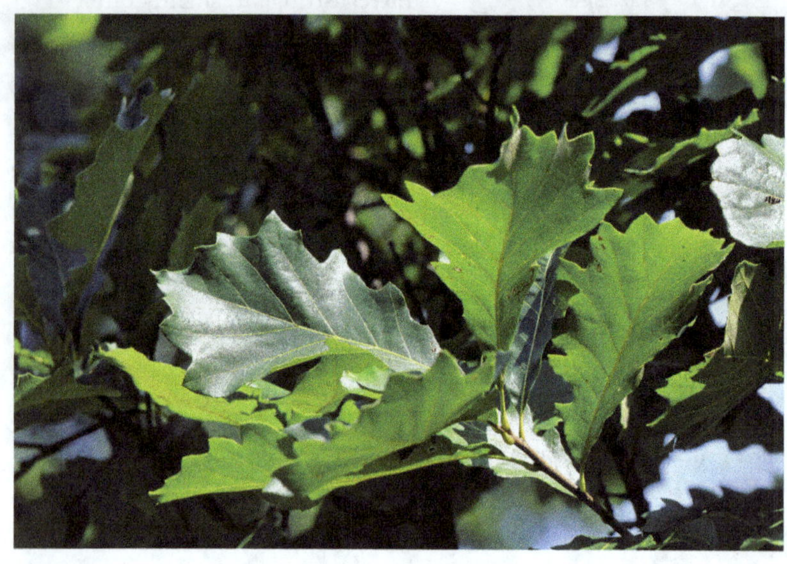

#28 – Oat Seed (Wild Oats, Oatstraw)

Avena Sativa

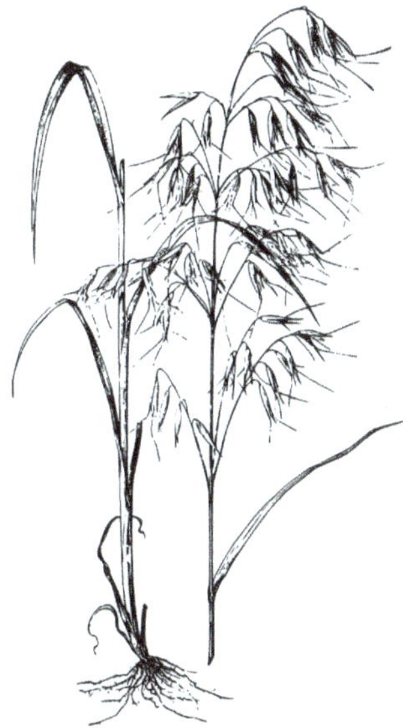

Parts Used: fresh, young oat seeds

Temperature: neutral

Taste: sweet

Actions: tonic, sedative, nervine, adaptogenic

Preparation and Dosage: Avena Sativa is best when taken as tea or mixed in another tincture as the adaptogenic component. Take a Standard Infusion by combining 1 tablespoon of the fresh herb or one teaspoon of the dried herb in 1 cup of boiling water. Please refer to the recipe section for further instructions.

Contraindications: This is a very mild herb. Follow the Standard Dosage instructions.

Habitat: Oat Straw or Avena Sativa is very easy to find in open sunny meadows. It has a long stalk that can grow up to 4 ft tall (1.2 m). You will discover smaller stems at the top of the stem with long pointed pods at the end. Harvest the pods in early spring.

Common uses: Oat Seed or Oatstraw is a classic nervine tonic. Oatmeal has a similar quality. It builds energy while reducing stress and is ideal for aging due to its tonic, nervine and demulcent qualities. It is beneficial for combating different addictions, including tobacco addiction, cannabis addiction, and even opium addiction. It uplifts you when you feel exhausted. Therefore, it helps with all the symptoms of burnout like anxiety, insomnia, weakness, fatigue, and exhaustion. Avena Sativa is exceptionally high in calcium and magnesium, two indispensable vitamins for supporting the central nervous system. It restores adrenal function.

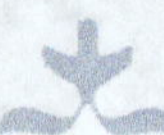

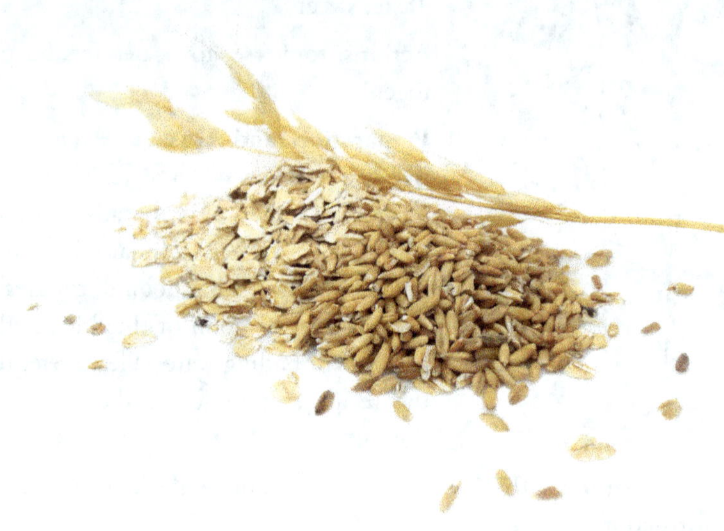

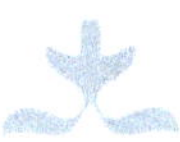

#29 – Pine

Pinus Sylvestris, sources: (1) (9)

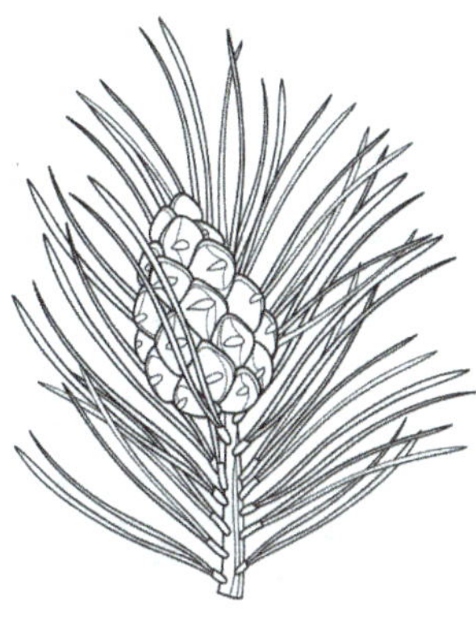

Parts Used: needles, buds.

Temperature: warming

Taste: bitter, sour

Actions: anti-inflammatory, stimulating, tonic, regenerates adrenals

Preparation and Dosage: Make an infusion using 1 cup of boiling water and ¼ cup of chopped pine needles. Take 3 cups daily, particularly for inflammation or fatigue.

Contraindications: Follow the directions when consuming this herb. There are no known side effects. There are over 60 species of pine trees. Most of them are edible. The most common in the US besides the Scotch pine are Eastern White Pine (Pinus strobus), Western White Pine (Pinus Monticola) and Sugar Pine (Pinus lambertiana). All edible pine needles have the same quality. All varieties of the Ponderosa Pine, the Yew tree and the Norfolk Island Pine are not edible. However, these pines are not nearly as common.

Habitat: The Scotch Pine is a coniferous tree that grows in Europe and Asia's cool, mountainous regions. It reaches heights of up to one hundred feet. It is both frost-resistant and loves sunlight. You might want to wear gloves when harvesting the needles because you can get sap on your hands. Gather the darkest green needles you can find. The younger, the better; they are the richest in plant constituents.

Common uses: Pine needles contain a fair amount of vitamin C and are high in antioxidants. Pine is anti-inflammatory. The vitamin C content of Pine needles tends to vary from species to species, and the younger pines tend to contain more. However, the Eastern White Pine needles in a USDA Forest study yielded between 0.72 mg and 1.87 mg of ascorbic acid per gram. In one historical account of voyages from

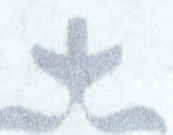

France to America, a French explorer Jaques Cartier in 1536, boiled Pine needles to remedy the scurvy of his crew. Guided by the local Iroquois, the crew recovered.

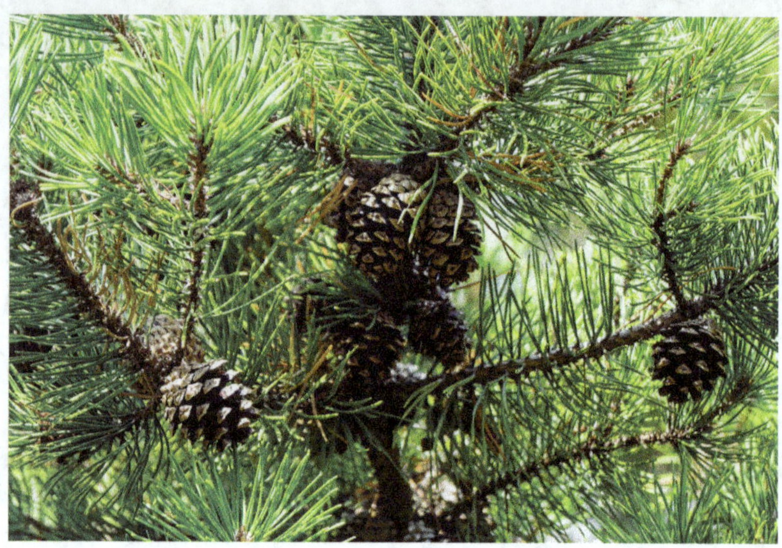

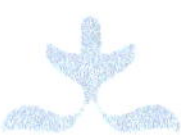

#30 – Plantain

Plantago Major, sources: (3) (6) (9) (12)

Parts Used: leaves or aerial parts

Temperature: cooling

Taste: slightly bitter

Actions: vulnerary, expectorant, demulcent, anti-inflammatory, astringent, diuretic, antimicrobial

Preparation and Dosage:

1. Take one teaspoon of the dried herb in 1 cup of boiling water three times daily.

2. Make a poultice by macerating two tablespoons of the leaves. Add one teaspoon of water.

3. Wash the leaves and add them to salads.

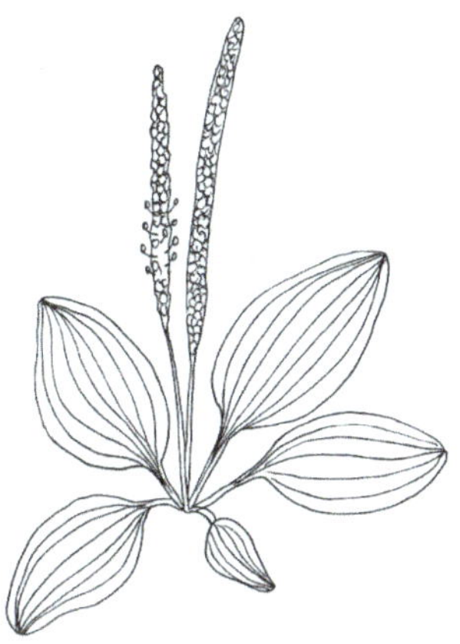

Contraindications: This gentle herb is very safe for children and the elderly. Please follow the recommended dosage.

Habitat: You will find Plantain in sandy, rocky, well-drained areas. It thrives in sunny conditions and often grows between other weeds on an ordinary lawn. Look for Plantain in vacant lots and waste areas or sunny meadows. There are two main types to identify. Plantago consists of broad leaves with equal parted leaves that fan out in groups or basal rosettes from the low base of the plant. The other variety, Ribwort, or long-leaved plantain has long, thin and very prominent ribbed leaves that rise up from the base. Both plants have a long stalk with seedlings that come up from the middle.

Common uses: Plantain was one of the most widely used Native American herbs. It is one of the easiest to find. The wide-leaf Plantain and its close relative Ribwort Plantain have valuable healing properties. Its power to extract toxins, poisons, and even small objects from the skin is remarkable. Plantain acts as a gentle expectorant. Its soothing, demulcent quality is perfect for inflamed and sore membranes. It works as a respiratory herb and can help soothe coughs and milder cases of bronchitis. It is ideal for children and more vulnerable populations. Its astringent qualities can help with diarrhea and hemorrhoids.

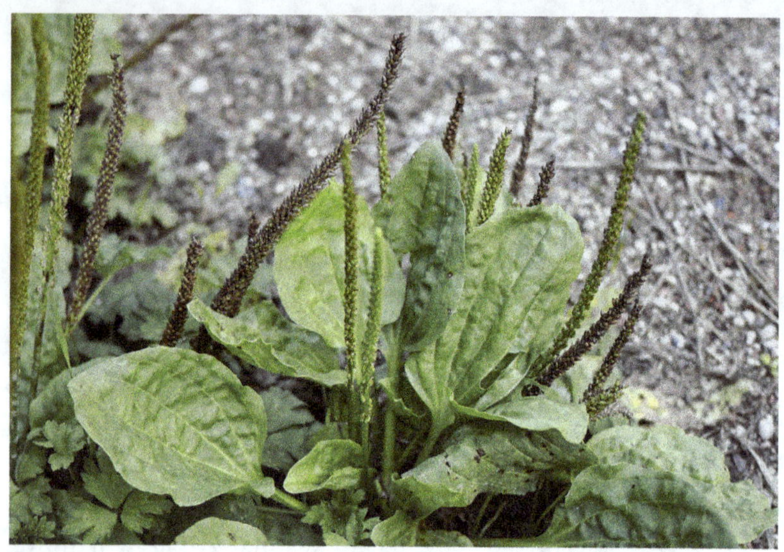

#31 – Red Clover

Trifolium Pratense, sources: (3) (6) (12)

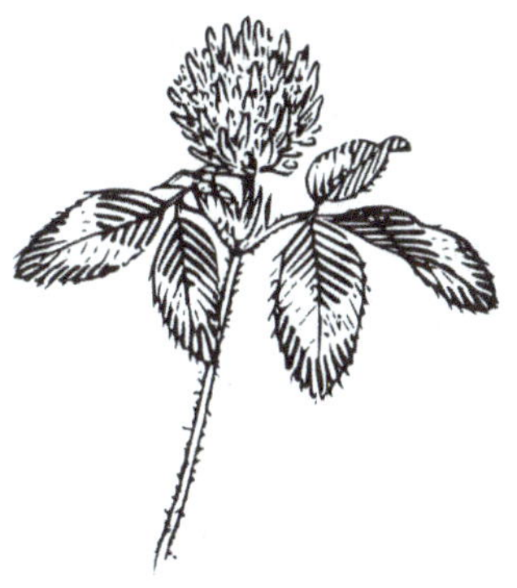

Parts Used: flower

Taste: aromatic, slightly bitter

Actions: alterative, expectorant, antispasmodic

Preparation and Dosage: Make a Standard Infusion of the dried flowers with 1 ½ teaspoon of the dried flower per 1 cup of boiling water. Take 3 cups daily.

Contraindications: Please follow the recommended dosage.

Habitat: Red Clover flowers thrive in open, sunny to partly shady meadows.

Common uses: Red Clover is one of the most valuable remedies for children's skin problems. It detoxifies the blood. When toxins are flushed out of the blood in general skin conditions often improve.

Its expectorant and antispasmodic actions make this remedy useful when treating coughs and bronchitis. It even treats whooping cough. It is effective when combined with other herbs to treat anemia. Europeans introduced this herb to the Americas, and it became widely used in native tribes for blood purification and stomach cancer.

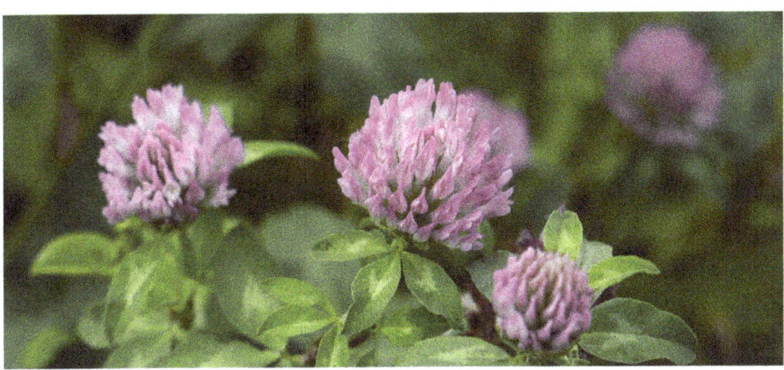

#32 – Roses (and Rosehips)

Rosa Canina, sources: (2) (3) (4) (17)

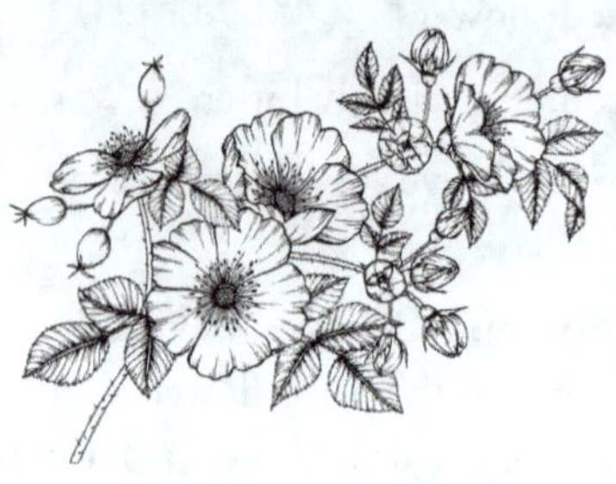

Parts Used: flower and rosehip.

Temperature: cooling

Taste: flower is aromatic, rosehips are sour and astringent

Actions: Rose: anti-inflammatory, adaptogenic, diaphoretic, anti-microbial, cardiotonic

Rosehips: nutritive, adaptogenic, astringent, tonic, vulnerary, anti-inflammatory

Preparation and Dosage: Rose petals do not make a good solitary tincture. They are too delicate, and the alcohol in the tincture diminishes the smell, its primary benefit. Rose is mild, so make an infusion with one tablespoon of the fresh petals per cup of boiling water or a rounded teaspoon of the dried. Take one cup three times daily. For Rosehip tea, put one teaspoon of the dried fruit in 1 cup of boiling water. Take three cups daily.

Contraindications: Both Rose and Rosehips are mild herbs with no known side effects.

Habitat: Wild Roses grow almost anywhere. Sometimes the bushes are pretty low to the ground. Roses resist pests and grow in open meadows, ravines, and open woods. The Rugosa Rose often grows near the oceanside and in fields.

Common uses: Rose is an ideal remedy for grief, shock, and trauma. It shifts someone from a mild or deep depression to an uplifted state.

Holly Bellubuono, an herbalist, tells a story of a traditional native midwife in Mexico who was assisting a difficult, high-risk birth. The mother, exhausted from pushing, lost the strength and the will to push the baby out of the birth canal. The midwife went out into the yard into a grove of Roses. She quickly gathered as many petals as she could

and brought them inside. She scattered the petals on a bedsheet and wrapped the traumatized mother up in it. Soon, the potent smell surrounded the exhausted new mother. She found the will to push, and the baby was delivered.

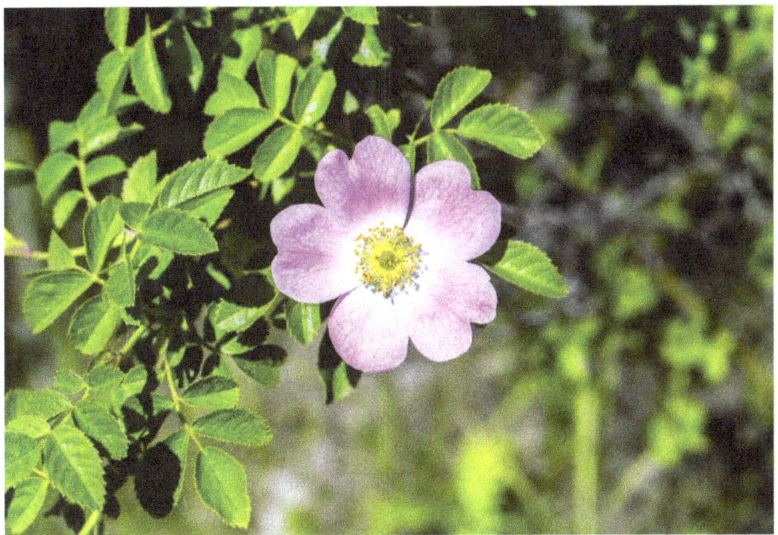

#33 – Rosehips

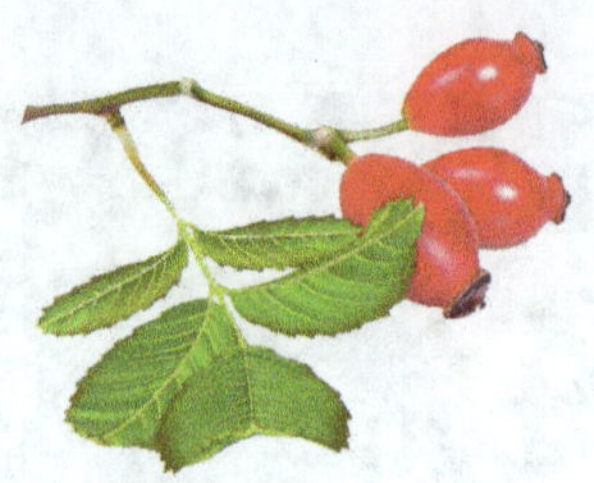

Many people have a Rosebush in their yard and yet are unaware that after the Rose fades away, a marvelous reddish bulb appears in its place that has excellent medicinal value.

Rosehips contain 4% vitamin C. The synergistic components of Rosehips maximize Vitamin C absorption. Rosehips scavenge free radicals with their antioxidant capabilities. They are anti-inflammatory, stabilize collagen, and help heal wounds and have been known to reduce tumors. Rosehips elevate the white blood cell count, enhancing immunity.

Northern Native American tribes found multiple uses for Rosehips. They extracted the juice and stored the herb for winter sustenance. Rosehip tea provided a perfect ear, nose, and throat remedy for children and the elderly. The tea is so powerful that it would strengthen childbearing women, thus facilitating delivery. Rosehips were often used for decorations and to bring good luck.

#34 – Rosemary

Rosemarinus Officinalis, sources: (17)

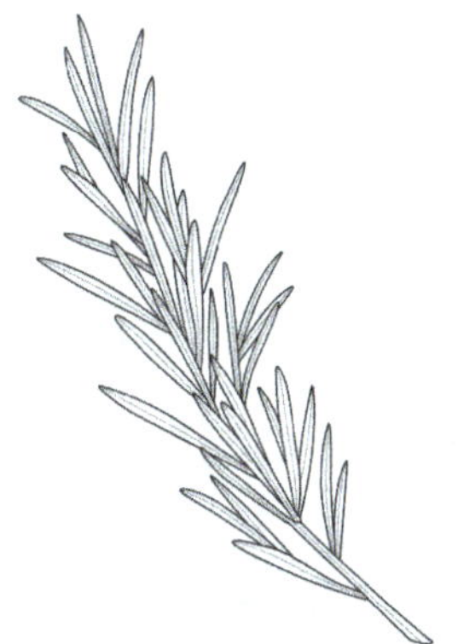

Parts Used: Leaves and stems

Temperature: warming

Taste: aromatic, bitter, pungent

Actions: rubefacient, adaptogenic, antidepressant, carminative, antimicrobial, hepatoprotective, anticarcinogenic, emmenagogue, antibacterial, antidiabetic, stimulates hair growth, improves memory, cephalic (relates to the head)

Preparation and Dosage: Make a Standard Infusion. Take one teaspoon of the dried herb in 1 cup of boiling water three times daily.

Contraindications: Please follow the recommended dosage. This herb is hypertensive and might raise blood pressure. Please use it with caution if you have a long and severe history of high blood pressure.

Habitat: The name Rosemary comes from the Latin word Ros Marinus meaning "the rose of the sea." It has an ancient Mediterranean origin. You will recognize it by the unmistakable aroma. You can identify its needles, resembling a miniature version of green balsam fir trees.

Common uses: It is not surprising that most Native American tribes viewed Rosemary as sacred. Besides ceremonial and ritual use, Rosemary is a stimulant for the circulatory system. It is warm and pungent, brings blood to the skin's surface and is helpful for musculoskeletal and neurological pain. Rosemary is an essential herb because it can alleviate mental and physical distress. Its combination of attributes makes it a wonderful cardiotonic herb in cases of weakness and fragility. Rosemary will calm and tone the digestive system, particularly a cranky digestive system that suffers from nervous debilitation.

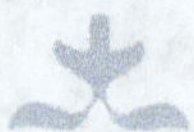

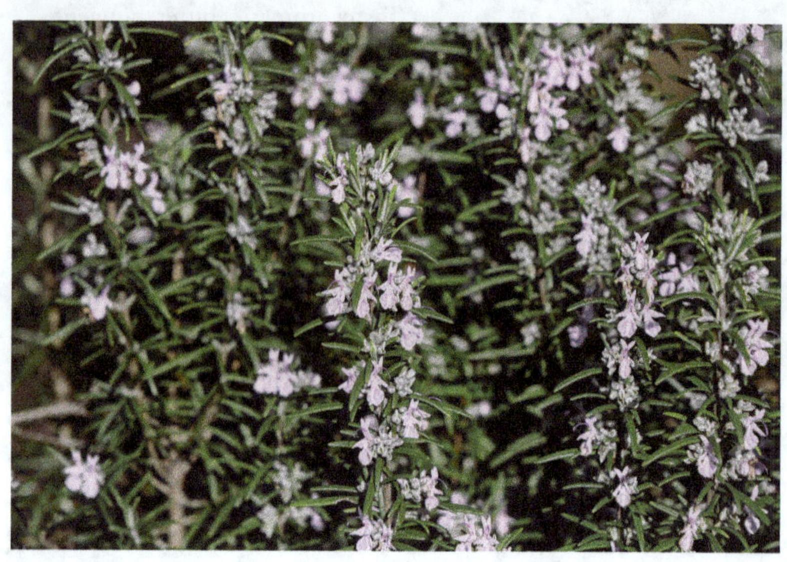

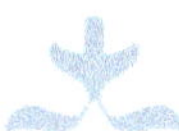

#35 – Sage

Salvia Officinalis, sources: (3) (6) (8) (12)

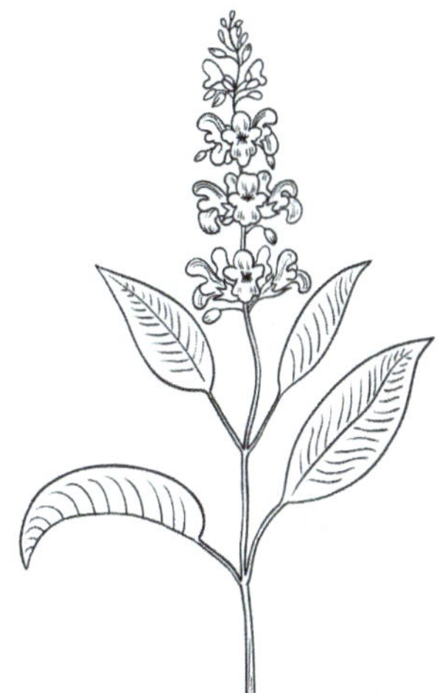

Parts Used: leaves

Taste: aromatic, slightly bitter

Actions: anti-inflammatory, adaptogenic, antispasmodic, astringent, antimicrobial, carminative, nervine

Preparation and Dosage: Infuse one teaspoon of the dried herb in 1 cup of boiling water. Just the aroma is a powerful healer for stress.

Contraindications: Sage is a gentle herb. Please follow the recommended dosage.

Habitat: Common Sage is an evergreen undershrub with silvery green leaves.

Common uses: Native Americans turned to Sage again and again for many common problems. Next to tobacco, it became the most sacred herb.

Sage decreases gas, bloating, diarrhea, intestinal spasms, and gastritis.

It is a superior herb for respiratory issues and a classic remedy for a simple sore throat. It acts on the oral cavity and the respiratory system to aid both laryngitis and pharyngitis. You can also use it for bleeding gums by swishing the tea around in your mouth for several minutes.

Sage's aroma assists with depression, anxiety, and mental exhaustion. It is a grounding herb and helps call the user back to the present moment. Much like Rosemary, it increases concentration and memory while decreasing fatigue. Native American healers used Sage poultices for menopause and any type of breast infection or impacted breasts due to mastitis.

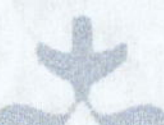

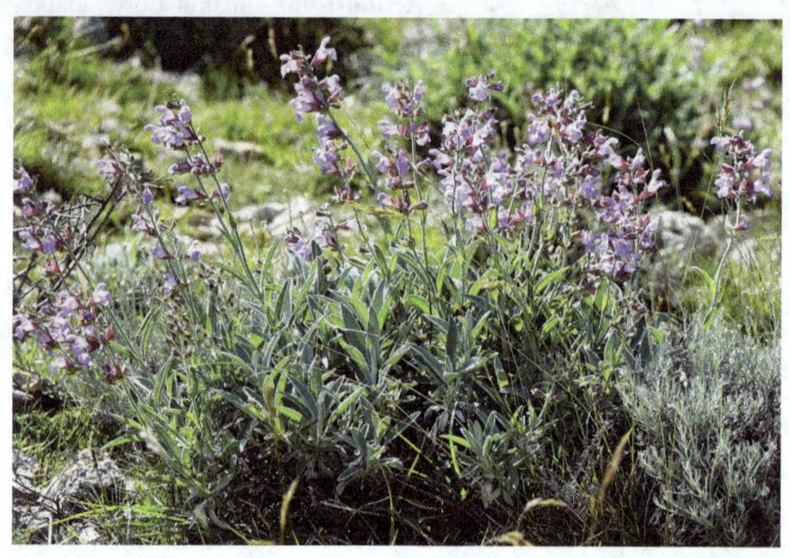

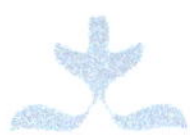

#36 – Saw Palmetto

Serenoa Repens, sources: (5) (6) (17)

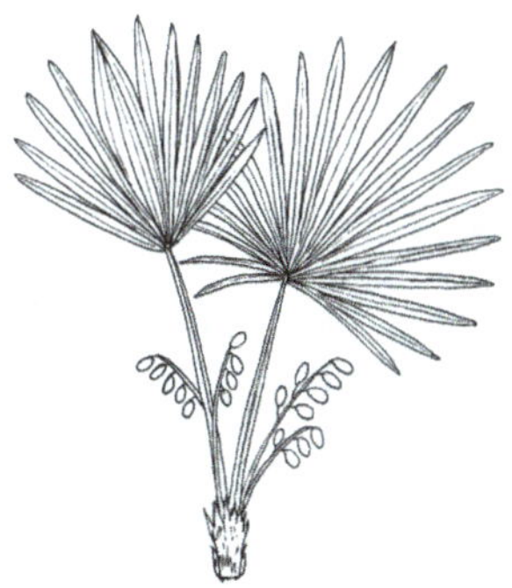

Parts Used: Berry

Taste: slightly sweet

Actions: anti-inflammatory, nutritive, adaptogenic, reproductive organ tonic, anti-tumor, cellular regeneration

Preparation and Dosage: Standard tea dosage applies. Take one teaspoon of the dried berry in one cup of boiling water three times daily. Pills from the powder are an option. Order from a reputable company. The standard dose is usually 500mg three times daily for most herbs. However, this varies. Discuss with your practitioner.

Contraindications: Please follow the recommended dosage.

Habitat: A Common palm that grows along the Atlantic shores from Florida to South Carolina and Louisiana. The dark red berries are the size of olives and are edible.

Common uses: Traditional Native American uses included using leaves for thatched huts and to stuff mattresses. The berries are profoundly nutritive and provide adaptogenic restoration at many levels. They seem to restore damaged reproductive organs in both males and females. Saw Palmetto is a tonic herb for the genital and urinary system.

Interestingly the berry is a sedative, nervine, and expectorant. Saw Palmetto restores exhausted libido. It is helpful for couples who are trying to conceive. It decreases impotence, encourages breast growth, and initiates the menstrual cycle. This plant, remarkably, assists with muscular development overall.

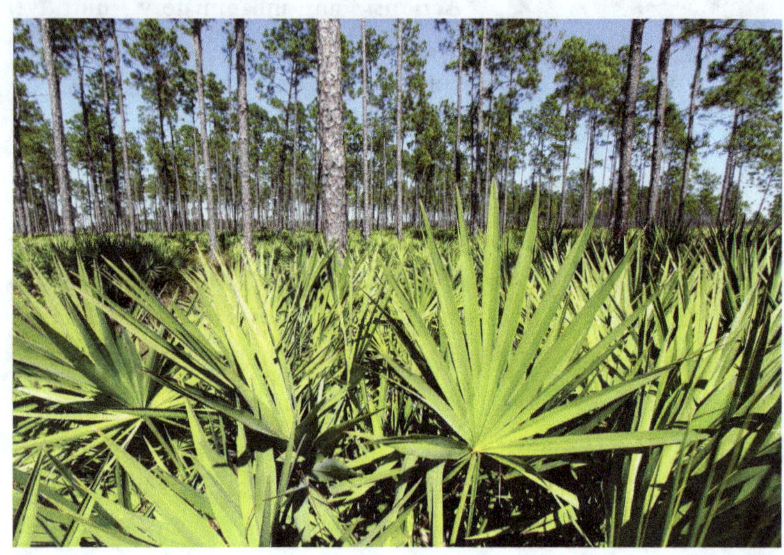

#37 – Uva Ursi

Arctostaphylos Uva-Ursi, sources: (3) (6) (12)

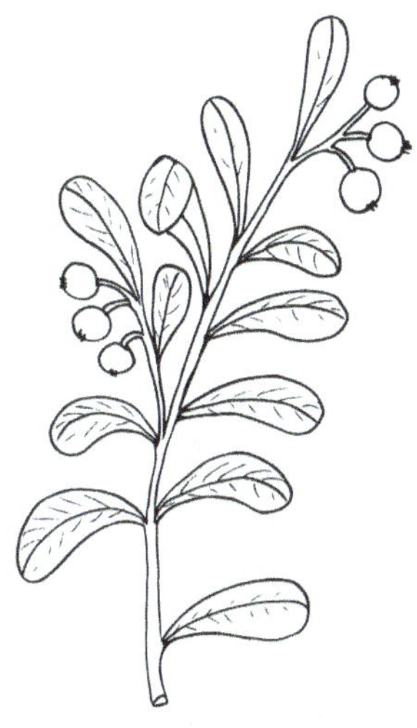

Parts used: leaves

Taste: bitter, astringent

Actions: diuretic, urinary, antiseptic, astringent

Preparation and Dosage: Place one teaspoon of the dried herb in one cup of boiling water. Take three cups daily.

Contraindications: Uva Ursi is a very astringent and drying herb. Its strength means it is effective, however you may want to consult with a practitioner prior to using it. They will provide an alternative. Uva Ursi can cause liver toxicity in overdose cases, particularly in people who have difficulty metabolizing acids. Do not take this herb if you are pregnant.

Habitat: Uva Ursi is evergreen and grows into the early winter months. Look for a shrub that is low to the ground. It often spreads on dry or rocky soil. You will see it trailing on stumps and over other plants. Bearberries have small red berries that appear in the spring that bears like to eat.

Common uses: Uva Ursi is used chiefly for urinary tract infections, including cystitis. It is also used for blood in the urine due to urinary tract infections or UTIs. It will strengthen the bladder and also subdue a mild kidney infection. An astringent tea from the dried leaves relieves constipation.

When the Algonquin tribe harvested this plant, they used the berries to control sexually transmitted diseases. They called Uva Ursi, 'Kinnikinnick' a term for tobacco substitutes because they would dry and smoke the plant.

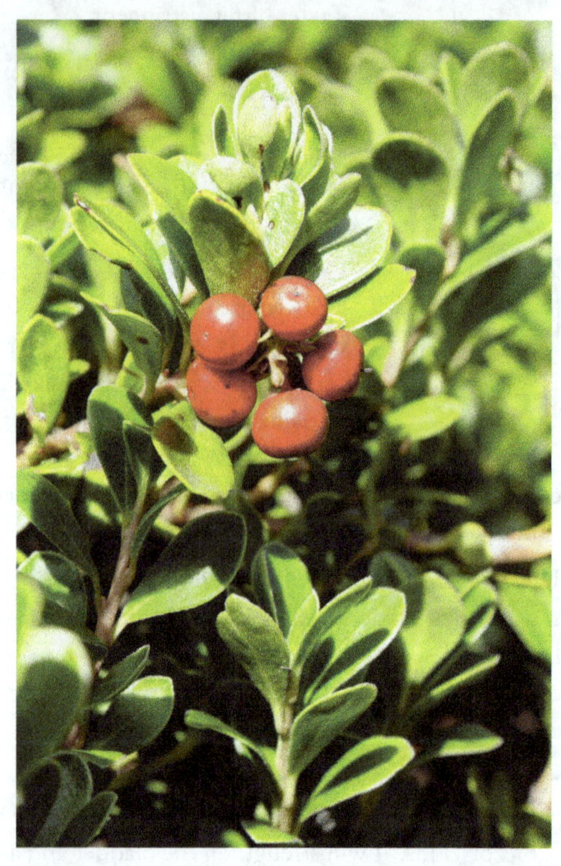

#38 – White Willow

Salix Alba, sources: (3) (6) (15)

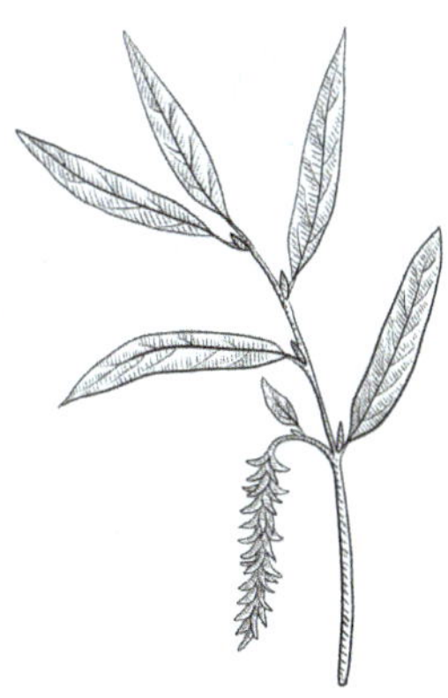

Parts Used: bark

Temperature: cooling

Taste: bitter

Actions: anti-inflammatory, antispasmodic, analgesic, sedative, antipyretic

Preparation and Dosage: Standard tea dosage applies to 1 teaspoon of the dried bark in one cup of boiling water three times daily. Taking the tea before bed reduces painful inflammation and promotes deeper sleep.

Contraindications: Please follow the recommended dosage.

Habitat: Its thin branches flow from the top, almost like a head of human hair. You will find this tree in bogs, open, damp, lowland wooded areas, or frequently at the edge of a pond. The leaves are swordlike with a grey-green color on top and a silvery-white color underneath. The other species also contain salicylic acid, but not as much as the White Willow. As the reader may recall, Meadowsweet also contains salicylic acid, but less than White Willow does.

Common uses: White Willow primarily reduces pain and inflammation. Traditional practitioners knew they could depend on it because they treated fevers with it consistently. That *which diminishes inflammation will also facilitate a fever.* Central to Northern tribes used Willow Bark frequently for pain relief. If time did not permit harvesting the bark and preparing a tea, they simply chewed on a medium-sized piece of bark for relief.

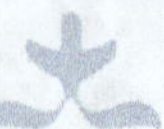

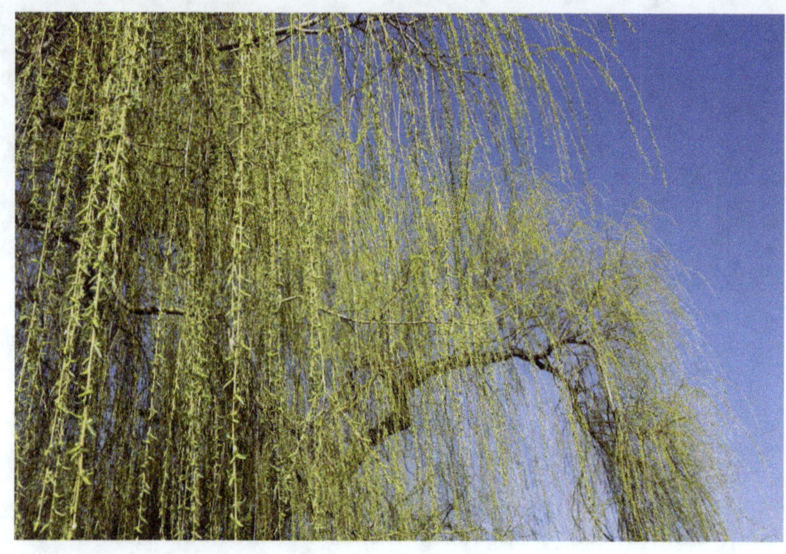

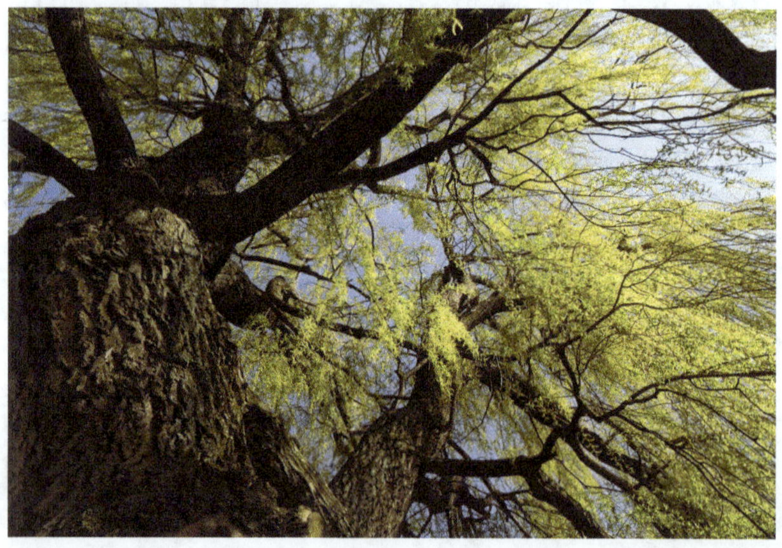

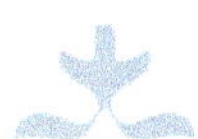

#39 – Yarrow

Achillea Millefolium, sources: (3) (4) (6) (8) (12)

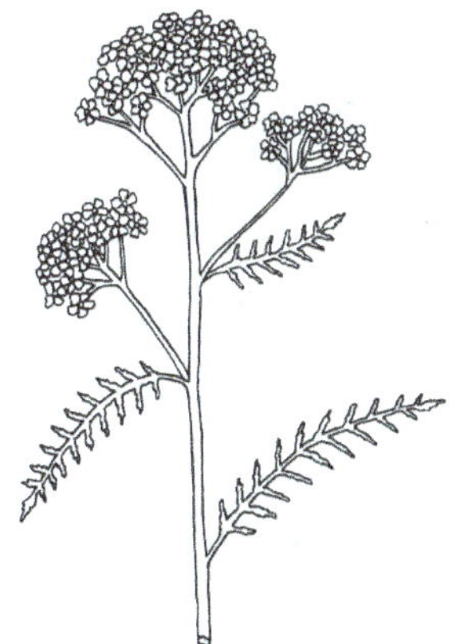

Parts used: aerial parts

Taste: bitter

Actions: diaphoretic, hypotensive, astringent, anti-inflammatory, diuretic, antimicrobial, alterative, hypotensive

Preparation and Dosage: Place 1 to 2 teaspoons of the dried herb in one cup of boiling water. Strain and take one cup three times daily.

Contraindications: Please follow the recommended dosage.

Habitat: Yarrow leaves are delicate and fernlike; the stems are pretty strong. The white, pink, or yellow flowers cluster at the top of the plant and the end of the side stems. The white flower variety works best for medicinal purposes. Yarrow grows in open meadows that are sunny and well-drained.

Common uses: Yarrow is a superior diaphoretic for lowering fevers and controlling coughs. It is very suitable for children and the elderly. Please recall this important feature during cold, cough, and flu season. The gentle herb is a steady companion for all in the family.

It also lowers blood pressure by simultaneously stimulating and toning the blood vessels. A simple poultice with Yarrow applied to a wound will stop bleeding. Native American tribes widely utilized Yarrow.

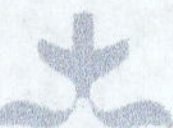

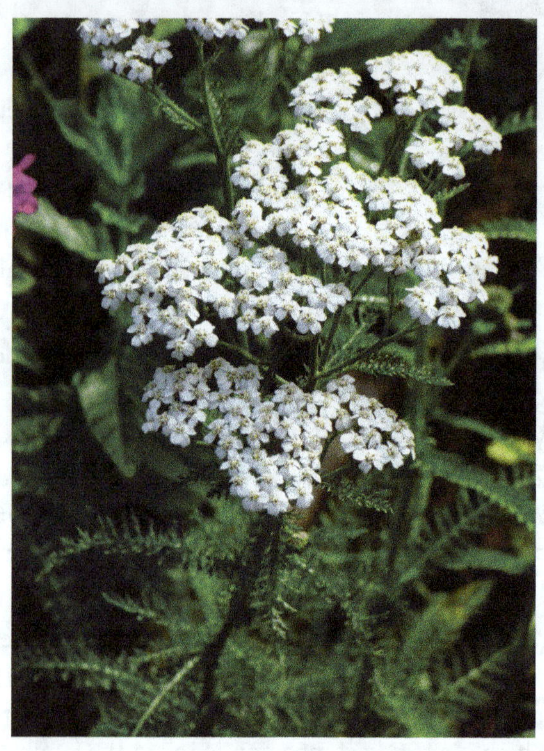

#40 – Yellow Dock

Rumex Crispus, sources: (3) (6) (12)

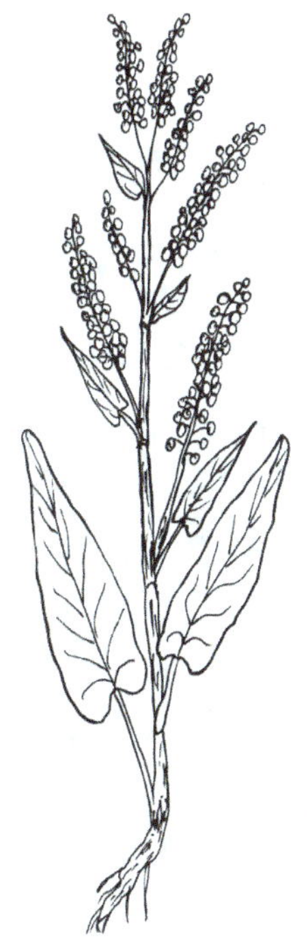

Parts Used: root

Temperature: cooling

Actions: alterative, cholagogue, blood tonic, astringent

Preparation and Dosage: Use the Standard Decoction of the roots to make the tea. Use one teaspoon of the dried root per cup of boiling water.

Contraindications: Use the Yellow Curly Dock roots, not the leaves, on this variety.

Habitat: Common in your backyard, shady meadow areas, and near riverbeds, first-year Yellow Dock will appear with oval leaves and 3" (7.5 cm) or stems with red veins close to the ground.

Common uses: Yellow Dock root is a beneficial herb for imbalances resulting from excessive liver and colon heat. It clears liver congestion and is a mild purgative for the large intestine. Indeed, it does have a laxative effect, but its star quality rests in treating anemia. As Cherokee tribes have shown, the root is your blood-building ally. Many Native American tribes across the Northern and Central areas of the U.S. used the leaves for sustenance, just like spinach. The Dakota made poultices from the leaves to heal wounds, and the Dakota, Cheyenne, and Blackfoot tribes used the fresh root to treat rheumatism. The Iroquis mashed the root and applied it to soothe hemorrhoids.

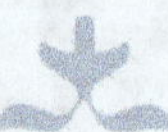

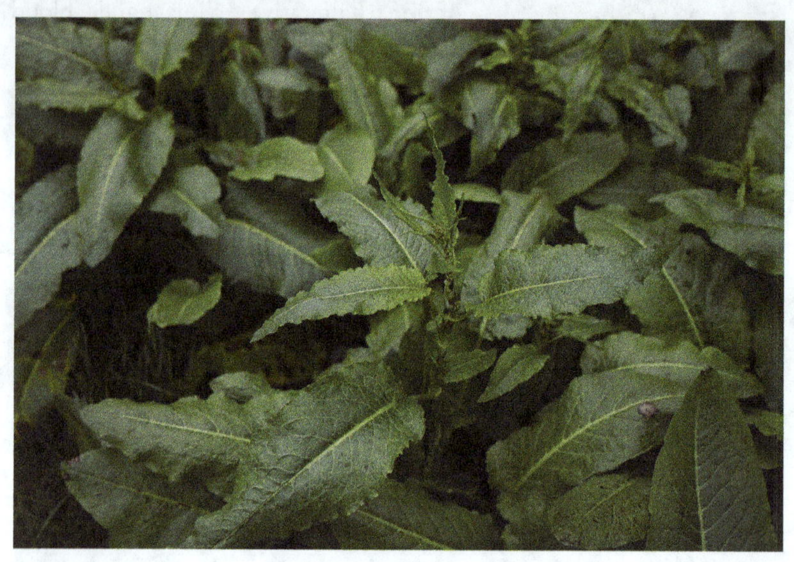

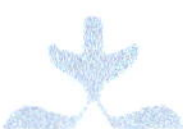

#41 – Yerba Santa (The Good Herb)

Eriodictyon Californicum

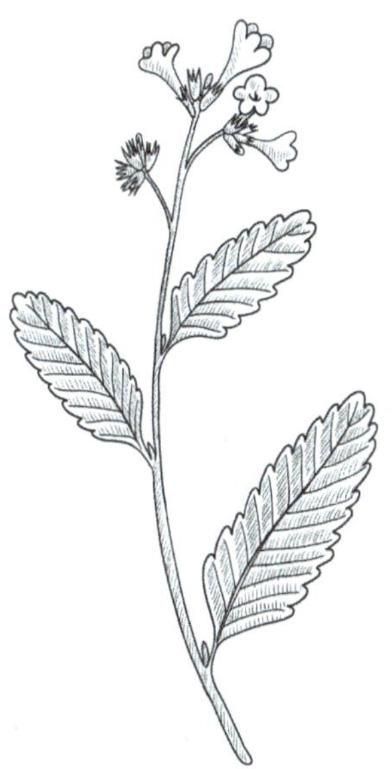

Parts used: leaves

Taste: slightly pungent, bitter

Actions: expectorant, carminative, alterative, sialogogue (promotes saliva), anti-inflammatory, vulnerary

Preparation and Dosage: Standard tea dosage applies. Place one teaspoon of the dried leaf in 1 cup of water. Take this three times daily.

Contraindications: Please follow the recommended dosage.

Habitat: Often, one will find this herb in Chaparral patches. Although not featured in this book, Chaparral is a pungent and astringent natural antibiotic that is more common in warmer western climates. Occasionally you can find Yerba Santa in a woodland area.

When you gather these leaves, smell them. They are reminiscent of an artificial cherry smell, for instance, in a cough drop.

Common uses: Also known as 'Holy Herb' or 'Mountain Balm,' Yerba Santa is an herb for upper respiratory congestion. Most tribes of the Pacific Northwest and the Cahuilla and Serrano Indians have gathered and used this plant for centuries. It is a bitter herb and an alternative, or liver cleanser, so while it expels mucus from your chest, it will also clear congestion in the liver. Yerba Santa also strengthens the spleen. The roots make an excellent poultice for rheumatism and arthritis.

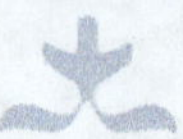

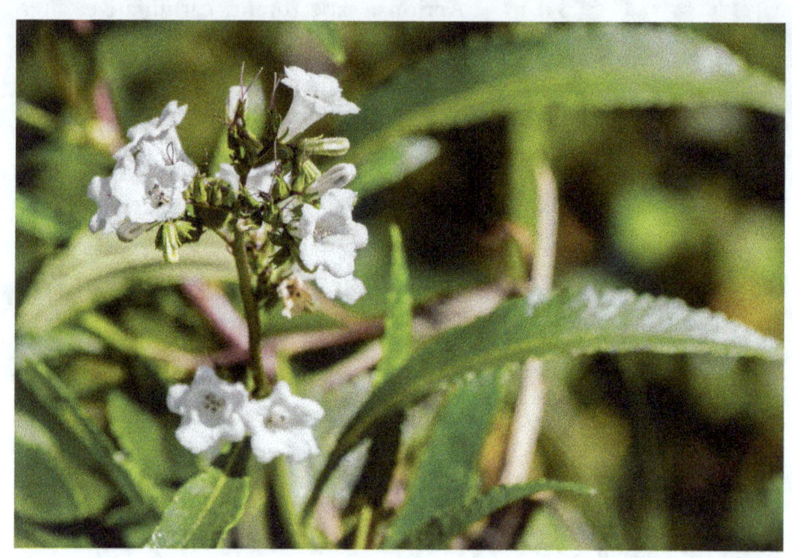

Sources

(4)   Barnes, R. L and Berry, Charles R. "Seasonal Changes in Carbohydrates and Ascorbic Acid and White Pine and Possible Relation to Tipburn Sensitivity" Res. Note SE-124. Asheville, NC: U.S. Department of Agriculture, Forest Service, Southeastern Forest Experiment Station, V 124, 1969, p.4

(5)   Bellebuono, Holly, "Women Healers of the World: The Traditions, the History, and the Geography," New York City: Skyhorse Publishing, 2014.

(6)   Gladstar, Rosemary, "The Art and Science of Herbalism," Vermont: Sage Mountain Publications, 2014.

(7)   Green, Matthew, "The Native American Healer Reviving The History of Her Ancestors," Interview with Linda Black Elk, Minnesota Public Radio, December 31, 2018

(8)   Hatter, Ila, Interview with #1 Snowbird Cherokee Elder "Mandy" Talks Herbal Medicine with Ila Hatter — YouTube, June 19, 2011.

(9)   Hoffman, David FNIMH, AHG, "Herbs for Healthy Aging: Natural Prescriptions for Vibrant Health" Vermont: Healing Arts Press, 2014. (See: Sarsaparilla)

(10)   Homewytewa, Theodora, "Naturally Occurring Plants Used On The Hopi Indian Reservation for Medicine and Food," National Proceedings: Forest and Conservation Nursery Associations, Utah: USDA Forest Service, 1999-2001.

(11)   Kreiger, Diane, "USC Pharmacist Uncovers Healing Powers of Native Plants," USC Trojan Family, Winter 2014

(12)   The Ladybird Johnson Wildflower Center, Plant Database, Seen on: Arctostaphylos uva-ursi (Kinnikinnick) | Native Plants of North America (*www.wildflower.org*), January 25, 2022.

(13)   Native American Indian Medicine, Legends of America, Seen on: Native American Medicine – Legends of America, January 24, 2022. *https://www.legendsofamerica.com/na-medicine/*

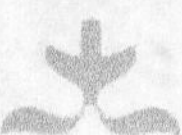

(14) Shaeffer, Elizabeth, "Dandelion, Pokeweed, and Coltsfoot: How the early settlers used plants for food, medicine and in their home," Dandelion, Addison-Wesley: Massachusetts, 1972.

(15) Tierra, Michael, L.Ac., OMD, "The Way of Herbs," New York: Pocket Books, 1998.

(16) Nafiseh Shokri Mashhadi, Reza Ghiasvand, Gholamreza Askari, Mitra Hariri, Leila Darvishi, and Mohammad Reza Mofid, "Anti-Oxidative and Anti-Inflammatory Effects of Ginger in Health and Physical Activity: Review of Current Evidence" International Journal of Preventive Medicine, 2013 Apr; 4(Suppl 1): S36–S42., Seen on: *https://www.ncbi.nlm.nih.gov/pmc/articles/PMC3665023/*

(17) University of Vermont Tree Profiles, Black Tupelo, Omeka@ CTL | UVM Tree Profiles: Black Tupelo: Cherokee Medicinal Use, Seen: January 23, 2022.

(18) Vassey, Christopher N.D., "Natural Remedies for Inflammation," White Willow," Vermont: Healing Arts Press, pp.81-82

(19) Watkins, Helen, "Devil's Club" Traditional Uses by the Tlingit Native American tribal elders of Alaska, April 1, 2016, Seen on: *https://www.youtube.com/watch?v=DyUssKc2TLQ*, January 22, 2022.

(20) Yance, Donald R., C.N., MH, R.H. (AHG), "Adaptogens in Medical Herbalism" Vermont: Healing Arts Press, 2014.

(21) Devil's Club, pp. 406-407 Taken from J. Tai, S. Cheung, S. Cheah, et al., "In vitro antiproliferative and antioxidant studies on Devil's Club Oplopanax horridus," Journal of Ethnopharmacology 6(3) 1982: pp.339-353.

- See profile on Ginger.
- See profile on Ginseng.
- See profile on Rosehips.
- See profile on Rosemary.
- See profile on Saw Palmetto.

(22)   United States Department of Agriculture, "Edible Seeds and Grains of California Tribes and the Klamath Tribe of Oregon," Phoebe Apperson Hearst Museum of Anthropology Collections, University of California, Berkeley (fs.fed.us), August 2012.

(23)   USDA Forest Service, Boise, Heartleaf Arnica, Seen on: Boise National Forest — Nature & Science (usda.gov)

(24)   American Society for Clinical Oncology, Memorial Sloan Kettering, June 25, 2016. Seen on: Black Cohosh — The ASCO Post, (*www.ascopost.com*)

(25)   American Indian Health and Diet Project, Food Indigenous to the Western Hemisphere, Sarsaparilla (www.ku.edu)

(26)   Utah State University, "Horsetail" Seen on: *https://extension.usu.edu/rangeplants/forbsherbaceous/horsetail#*, January 27, 2022.

(27)   Polizzi, Nick, Interview with Dennis Martinez, " 2 Sacred Medicine Trees of North America", Seen on: 2 Sacred Medicine Trees of North America — The Sacred Science The Sacred Science, January 27, 2022.

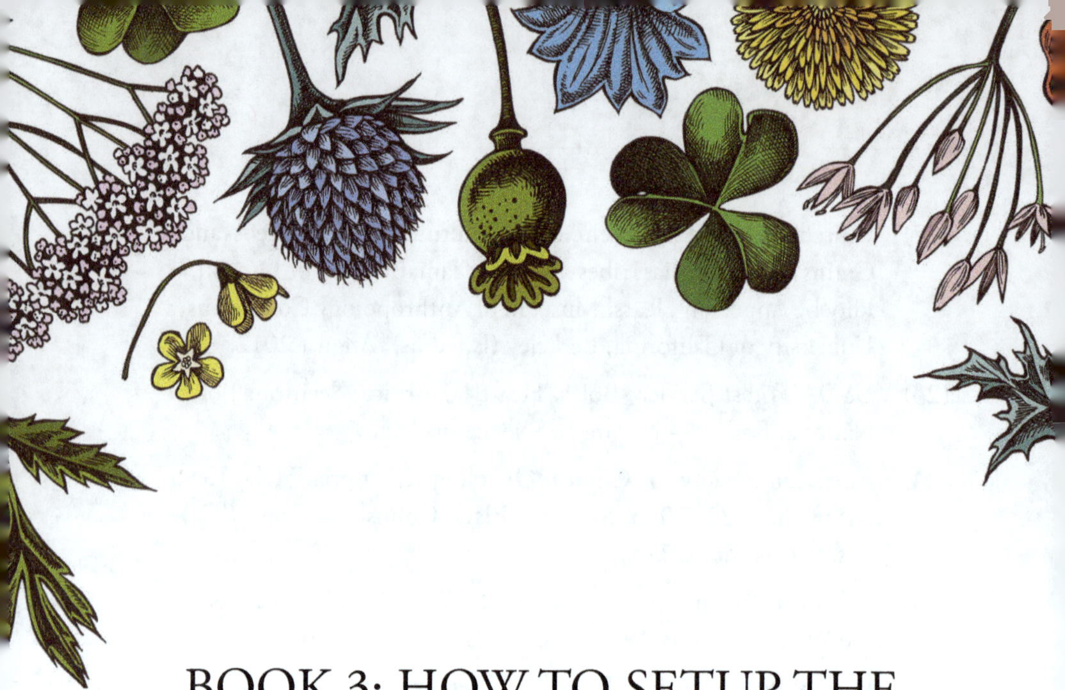

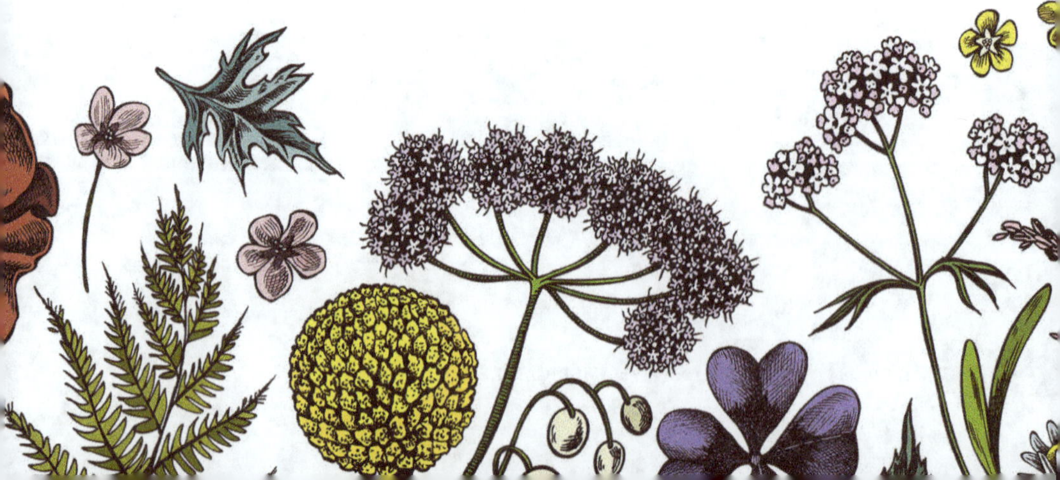

BOOK 3: HOW TO SETUP THE APOTHECARY TABLE THAT MATCHES YOUR NEEDS

"Honor the sacred. Honor the Earth, our Mother. Honor the Elders. Honor all with whom we share the Earth: Four-leggeds, two-leggeds, winged ones, Swimmers, crawlers, plant and rock people. Walk-in balance and beauty."

—Native American Elder

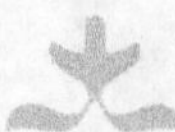

9   Tools and techniques for Making Your Own Herbal Medicine

9.1   Supplies needed for preparing herbal formulas

Stocking your supplies to make remedies before you start collecting herbs is important. You will feel unprepared if you end up with an herb without the objects necessary for preparation.

Here is a list of what you need (see also the illustrations below):

1. Cheesecloth to strain your remedies — One main benefit of cheesecloth is that you can squeeze it when you strain it to remove the core of the botanical extracts. Note: in a pinch, you can also use a coffee filter.

2. Mortar and pestle for making spice blends.

3. An assortment of funnels.

4. Clean, sanitized jars (2oz, 4oz, 8oz and 16oz) A variety of jars means that no matter what amount of an herb you procure, you are ready to store it properly.

5. A double boiler to condense some of your formulas and create salves. if you don't have one at home then just put a bowl in a cooking pot.

6. Parchment paper or clean paper bags to dry your herbs on

7. String to tie your herbs and hang them to dry.

8. Cotton or flannel cloths (a dishtowel works well) to cut up and use for poultices and compresses.

9. A few ounces of beeswax to make salves.

10. At least 12 ounces of olive oil to make oil extractions and salves.

11. A basket or cloth bag to carry with you while you forage.

12. Two-ounce dropper bottles (brown or blue) to make your first tincture. Order a dozen to start. A two-ounce bottle will yield three doses of 1", or one dropper full, for about twenty-five days.

13. Optional: you can order tea bags online or you can simply strain your loose tea.

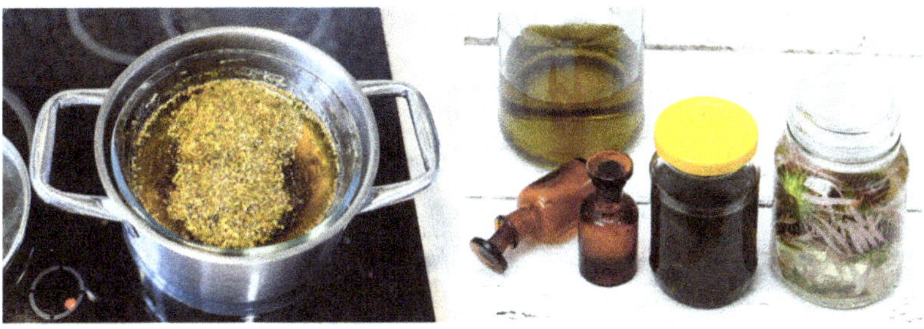

Picture left: Self-made 'double boiler' with bowl in a cooking pot.
Right: jars for storing herbs and herbal remedies.
Remember to store them at a dark, cool place.

9.2   Techniques to Harness the Power of Herbs

Many people are terrified at the thought of making their own medicine. This common fear can be alleviated by simply understanding what is involved in the process and getting to know the qualities of the plants themselves. You will be very encouraged to learn that overall, the risks of herbal medicine making are quite low. With all due respect, most master herbalists, herbal teachers, and a growing number of physicians are well aware of the fact that fewer lives have been harmed by herbs, than by the consequences of relying exclusively on pharmaceutical prescriptions.

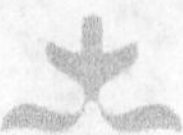

You already add medicinal spices to your food, you already make tea, and you may have followed your grandmother's advice about taking a natural remedy. Plus, just picking up this book shows you are eager to learn about natural healing. You are already qualified! Rest assured in the competence of our ancient teachers. Herbalism is both an art and a science, finely tuned over thousands of years.

We have to bear in mind that formulation techniques used today differ in some ways from traditional Native American preparations. In previous sections we have seen how they used teas, baths, and chewing the herb directly (e.g. chewing Willow Bark for pain relief or Greenbrier to reduce inflammation). Other common uses included poultices, compresses, and smoking the herb directly for ceremonial purposes.

Unless one uses the herb directly, herbs require a liquid menstruum, or medium, to break down their properties so the body can absorb them. One extracts the primary medicinal herbal components in so-called 'menstruums' that have different potency levels to harness the power of the herb.

Here are the main ones:

1. Water — is used for teas, steaming and baths, compresses, poultices, and oral swishes.
    Water as a menstruum is gentle and easily absorbed. Hot water breaks down herbal components.

2. Alcohol — for instance vodka, or another type of liquor used for tinctures kept in dropper bottles is a superior menstruum.
    Alcohol is advantageous because it breaks down the oils in herbs like tannins that contain valuable healing properties.

3. Vinegar — used in the same way as alcohol, to extract herbal properties to make tonics, administered by teaspoon.
    Vinegar is a useful medium because its extraction power is just a bit below alcohol but it contains other properties that optimize digestion.

4. Honey — is a good menstruum for children's formulas like syrups, administered by teaspoon.

5. Glycerin — is a good menstruum for children's formulas or for people who cannot tolerate alcohol tinctures, administered by teaspoon.

    Glycerin provides an alternative to honey, is tolerated by those who cannot have alcohol, and is inexpensive.

6. Oil — is used to extract herbal properties to make massage oils, and salves.

    Oil is advantageous because it allows people to make their own topical applications.

9.3   Water As a Menstruum

Infusions

Infusions are teas made with leaves and flowers. If you have made a delicious cup of tea at any point in your life, you are perfectly qualified to create infusions. The only difference is understanding how to administer the right medicinal dose.

The medicinal dosage of tea for a chronic condition is three cups a day. However, it is very tedious to make a cup at a time. Make three quarts of tea at time if you are taking a remedy for more than a week. Take your daily dose of three cups of your preferred tea and store the other two quarts in the refrigerator.

Making tea in advance is practical. If you are sick, you don't want to get in and out of bed all of the time and disturb your sleep, just to make tea.

Of all the remedies, teas are the easiest to make:

1. Boil your water, and put your herbs in a small pot for infusion.

2. Traditionally, one teaspoon of dried herb, or one tablespoon of chopped fresh herbs is required per cup of water. A storebought tea bag typically contains a teaspoon of a dried substance.

3. Cover your herbs with the boiled water and steep for 15 minutes. Hot water is your mentruum. It breaks down the components of an herb. Remember, heat creates movement so you are making

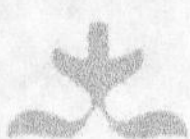

it possible for your herbs to move throughout your body and complete their actions.

4. Strain and store in a glass jar.

5. Infusions are bursting with life and therefore attract microorganisms! Make sure to discard your tea after storing it if it tastes fermented or smells spoiled.

Tea works with the body in a unique way. Our bodies are made of roughly 80% water. An herbal tea infusion is a remedy that balances the water content in your body. The medicinal tea ingredients carried in water flush unwanted bacteria, and toxins from various systems.

Infusions are bursting with organic life and therefore attract microorganisms! Make sure to discard your tea after storing it if it tastes fermented or smells spoiled. If you want, you can order muslin or paper tea bags to make your own tea bags.

Decoctions

Decoctions are similar to infusions, but they are required for a more sensitive medium like a bark, seed or a root. The proportions are the same, either 1 teaspoon of dried root, seed, or bark, or 1 tablespoon of fresh root, seed or bark per cup of water. Mint is a leaf so you will infuse it, while Ginger is a root, so you will decoct that.

1. Slowly simmer the decoction for twenty minutes. Add a little water at the end to make up for the evaporation.

2. Strain and store in a glass jar.

3. Teas made with barks or roots tend to last up to a week when refrigerated. Make one to three quarts at a time.

Herbal Steams/Epsom Salts Baths/Foot Soaks

Herbal steams with essential oils, herbal baths and herb foot soaks with hot water are important methods for clearing stagnation, reducing infection, for nourishment, and simple restoration.

Herbal Steaming

If an herb is aromatic, like mint leaves, roses or lemon balm you can make an infusion in a small pot and create a tent over your head with a towel to breathe in the aroma. Different herbs like mint for instance clear the nasal passages and also are sedative.

1. Chop 1 tablespoon of fresh leaves or roots and place them in 1 quart of boiling water.

2. Make a tent over your head with a hand towel and ***put your face at least a foot above the steam. You do not want to burn your skin.***

3. Inhale until the smell fades.

4. Dry your face off and cover up to prevent any exposure from the cold. Rest if needed.

5. Repeat this three to five times per day depending on the condition. If it is chronic three times is fine. If it is acute, five times may be required.

Herbal Baths

Soaking in an herbal bath is basically like drinking an enormous cup of tea (safely of course). Your skin is the largest organ in your body; it absorbs nutrients and also expels toxins through its pores. Baths are a time-tested form of healing and were utilized by native tribes.

For instance, to stop a child's diarrhea they would have placed the child in a small tub of blackberry leaf infused water. Absorbing the water through their skin in a hot tub was relaxing. It avoided the issue of trying to give a bitter tea to a child to ingest.

Prepare a bath using the following steps:

For a fresh herbal bath:

1. Take two cups of a chopped herb tied up in cheesecloth. Place this in 4 cups of boiling water. For leaves infuse for 15 minutes, for roots, seeds and bark decoct for 20 minutes.

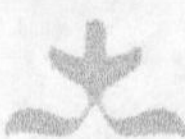

2. Cool and strain your tea.

3. Run your bath water.

4. Put the tea in your bath.

For a bath using essential oils:

1. Run a hot bath and put 15–20 drops of essential oil in the bath.

2. Swish it around with your hand to disperse it before you get in the bathtub.

3. Stay in the bath for at least fifteen minutes so that your skin can absorb the oils.

Don't use mint oil in the bathtub! It is too cooling and does not break down as well in the hot water so ironically it can also burn the skin.

Foot Soaks

A foot soak works in the same way as a bath and is tolerated more easily by those who cannot get into the bathtub.

1. Use ½ cup of chopped herbs.

2. Tie them in a square of cheesecloth.

3. Heat three-quart of water.

4. Find a suitable chair for the person to sit and place a towel on the floor in front of the chair.

5. Put the foot tub on the towel and fill it with hot water.

6. Place the three cups of herbal water that you have either infused or decocted into the tub.

7. A person can sit and relax here for up to a half-hour absorbing the herbal benefits.

8. Dry the feet and put on a pair of cotton socks to let the skin breathe.

9. Once or twice a day for a chronic condition should be enough.

Oral Swishes

Oral swishes are an excellent form of preventative dental care and maintenance. They can also help reduce canker sores, toothaches or any other sore in the mouth.

An **oral swish** occurs when you use a tincture or strong tea and continually swish it in your mouth to decrease inflammation and infection. Maybe you have already done this with simple warm salt water, for instance, to reduce an abscess. You will find a recipe for a Sage oral swish in this book.

1. Take 1" or tincture or 1 tablespoon of strong tea into the oral cavity. Tea or tincture will vary depending on the ailment you wish to treat.

2. Swish the liquid in the oral cavity but do not swallow it. Let it touch the inner surfaces of the mouth so it is absorbed.

3. After ten minutes, spit it out in the garbage.

Let the liquid soak into the oral tissues and follow up by drinking a glass of water after another ten minutes or so.

Compresses

Making a compress is a lot like making a cup of tea. However, you must have a square cotton or flannel cloth on hand for topical application.

1. Make a cup of tea with one cup of boiling water and 1 teaspoon of the chosen herb (for example, Ginger or Devil's Club to reduce inflammation)

2. Fold a flannel or cotton cloth into a square.

3. Strain the tea and pour it into a bowl.

4. When it has cooled down so you can touch it, soak the cloth in it. Make sure that it is still warm.

5. Ring out the cloth and apply to the affected area for twenty minutes. You can repeat this process three times a day, or repeatedly in acute cases of inflammation.

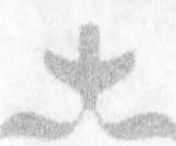

Poultices

A poultice is usually made from an herbal paste, a chopped and cooked herb, or in an emergency a quickly macerated herb. It is spread on an injury, ache or wound. You will hold this paste in place with a cloth. A poultice can pull infections and toxins from an affected area or heal a wound.

1. Prepare a half cup of herbs by the infusion or decoction method. Another example is baking soda in water to make a paste.

2. Strain and place on the affected area.

3. Cover with a flannel or cotton cloth and hold for twenty minutes. You can tie a band around the cloth to hold it in place.

4. Dry the area but do not scrape it. Let the herbal residue continue to soak in.

5. Reapply as needed depending on the condition.

9.4   Using Alcohol As A Menstruum

Tinctures

Tinctures are made with alcohol, vinegar, honey, and glycerin. Tinctures break the components of the herbs down and concentrate them, through the process of extraction. ***Extraction is the heart of formulating herbal remedies.*** Concentrated extractions release the components of herbal actions to enable healing.

Alcohol is uniquely effective at breaking down the components of an herb, releasing them into the menstruum. For those who cannot tolerate alcohol, like children of alcoholics, some tinctures in this book will be made with vinegar, honey, or glycerin.

This book teaches the simpling method and only gives a recipe for one more complex anti-viral formula. An alcohol tincture is the easiest way to make a remedy, besides making tea.

Using the simpling method you will cover your herbs in a glass jar with the menstruum you are using, Generally, it ends up balancing — a 50% to 50% ratio, herb/menstruum. If your herbs soak up the menstruum, simply add more alcohol to the top until it covers the herb. Do not add water to your tinctures or they will attract mold.

The simpling method has been practiced for thousands of years. A huge benefit is that if you find a remedy and make a batch of it, for less than fifty dollars a batch you will have enough remedy for six months at the chronic dose level.

People certainly have their preferences for the type of alcohol used. Mainly, it needs to be at least 60 proof in order to break down the herbs (primarily the oils, terpenes in them). Plain vodka is generally recommended, especially if you are just starting out. It is easy to work with, effective and has little taste.

1. Start with a clean jar. If your jars and lids are not clean, your medicine might acquire fungus or bacteria.

2. Put your herbs in the bottom and add your menstruum, in this case, alcohol over the herbs.

3. Close the jar and let this sit in a dark place, with a neutral temperature, for twenty-one days. (The twenty-one day waiting period is a traditional ancient practice.)

4. After twenty-one days, line a strainer with cheesecloth and strain your tincture into a bowl.

5. Gather the edges of the cheesecloth and twist them until you squeeze out the very last drop of your medicine. Those last drops contain the highest concentration of ingredients from your herbs.

6. Use a funnel or a vessel with a spout to pour your herbal liquid into a glass jar for storage.

7. Cap and store in a cool dark place. The mixture will store for several years or more.

Alcohol tinctures can be stored for the longest period of time. Consequently, they are convenient and cost-effective.

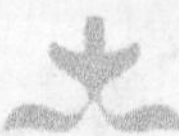

9.5 Using Vinegar, Honey or Glycerin As A Menstruum

Vinegar

Vinegar contains acetic acid and is a solvent and preservative like alcohol, only not quite as strong. You would follow the same simpling procedure using **vinegar** for tonic preparations.

The benefit of using vinegar is that it is non-toxic and tolerated by almost everyone. People who cannot drink alcohol can consume vinegar. It has excellent nutritional benefits; it restores your microbiome (the lining of your gut) and rejuvenates the health of the digestive tract. Vinegar has a slightly laxative effect.

Glycerin

Glycerin is used for children and in some cases for adults who cannot handle alcohol. It does not break down oils and resins as well as alcohol or vinegar. The tincturing process is different from the simpling method.

1. Dilute the glycerin with water by half 50% to 50%.

2. Cover your herbs with the diluted glycerin and strain after two to three weeks.

3. Store your syrup in a clean glass jar.

Honey

Honey as a menstruum is in a category alone. Sometimes referred to as an 'elixir', it is a powerful mentrum. It is a great way to deliver medicine to children, and those resistant to herbal preparations. There are two main ways to prepare medicine using honey.

1. You can soak certain herbs in honey by covering them with honey and letting them sit in a cool dark place for three weeks or longer. The honey, after a couple of weeks will break the herb-

al components down and extract them. For instance, you could make Ginger, Garlic or Rose elixir in this manner.

Or use the second method:

2. Infuse or decoct your herbs in a pot on the stove, cool, strain, and add the honey afterwards. An example of this method is Elderberry syrup, discussed in the recipe section.

9.6   Taking Herbal Powders

Making your own herbal pills is a time-consuming process. Purchasing pills is an option. Better yet, you can take the powder in a medium such as:

1. Yogurt

2. Pudding

3. Oatmeal

4. Juice

Standard dosage of herbal powders is 500mg three times daily. This varies, however, depending on the herbal substance.

500mg equals ½ teaspoon in general

One option is to place ½ teaspoon of herbal powder in a small cup, mix it with one of the choices listed above and swallow. You would do this three times daily for a chronic condition.

Adjust the child's dose as needed. Alternatively look at the herbal cookie recipe. It provides a more interesting way for your family take medicine. You can use the cookies preventatively to boost the immune system or when a child gets sick, if they can swallow them, as a 'treat'. Another tasty alternative is lozenges.

Herbal Powder in Lozenges as Herbal Medicine

You will be surprised how simple it is to prepare your own throat lozenges.

 HERBALIST'S GUIDE TO NATIVE AMERICAN REMEDIES

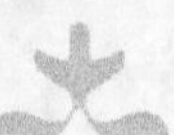

1. Prepare one ounce of Tragacanth (a natural gum you can order online) by melting it in 1 pint of boiling water.

2. After melting, soak the mixture for twenty-four hours.

3. The following day, beat the mixture to make it smooth.

4. Strain it through two layers of cheesecloth to make a mucilaginous liquid.

5. Add 1 tablespoon of brown sugar.

6. Add 2 tablespoons or more of the herbal powder you choose.

7. Put cornflour on a surface to roll out the paste.

8. Roll out the paste covering it with the cornflour.

9. Let it cool and then cut it into squares.

10. Store the lozenges in a tin or glass container.

Take the lozenges as needed depending on the amount of herbal powder in each lozenge.

9.7 Using Oil As A Menstruum

Oil Infusions (Oleolites)

When a plant is extracted in oil it is called an oleolite. Usually an oleolite will alleviate skin issues, including inflammation. It is always a good idea to keep an oil extraction handy for making your salves, for use as massage oil, or for aches and pains. If you use just the right ingredients, for instance roses, your oil extraction serves as a beauty product as well.

1. In a quart sized jar place 1 cup of your dried herb, or two cups of a fresh herb.

2. Cover the herb completely with whatever oil you choose (olive, almond, avocado, apricot are good choices)

3. Cover the jar with a lid.

4. Store in a cool, dark place for thirty to forty days. It takes a long time for oil extractions to finish. Oil is a very dense menstruum.

5. Shake the jar a couple of times a week to mix your ingredients.

6. After the extraction is finished, strain the oil into a strainer lined with cheesecloth that sits over a bowl.

7. After the oil drips through the cloth, gather the edges of the cloth and twist and squeeze all of the oil out into the bowl.

8. Pour the finished extraction into a glass jar.

9. Store in a cool, dark place. Oleolites have a fair degree of shelf stability and will last for a couple of years when stored properly.

Salves

Salves are applied topically, only. Many people turn to salves because if they contain anti-inflammatory herbs, they are an effective alternative to using NSAIDs[4] For salves, the oil extractions you make will be your menstruum.

Here is the general recipe for a salve:

1. Warm 1 cup of herbal extracted oil you have prepared in a double boiler.

2. Add ¼ cup of beeswax and stir until melted.

3. Pour into small jars or metal tins. Cap and store in a cool, dark place.

9.8   Aromatherapy

Aromatherapy began with the practice of smelling the plant itself. Just smelling a rose, or a pine tree, or rosemary bush has a healing effect. Aromatherapy involves using a very concentrated essence of the plants.

---

4   Non-steroidal anti-inflammatory drugs (NSAIDs) are medicines that are widely used to relieve pain, reduce inflammation including acetaminophen and ibuprofen.

   HERBALIST'S GUIDE TO NATIVE AMERICAN REMEDIES

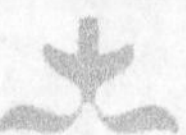

It is not an oleolation. An aromatic essential oil is much more concentrated. It takes thirty to fifty roses to produce one drop of rose essential oil! Two hundred and fifty pounds of lavender produce one pound of lavender essential oils. The underlying principle of aromatherapy is "less is more". Aromatherapy is a vast science in and of itself and it is not possible to go into depth in this book.

With just a few drops, a person can achieve powerful results, particularly when it comes to mood alteration and alleviating skin issues. European chemists refined the practice of aromatherapy through steam distillation although simple oil extractions have been used for hundreds of years.

Essential oils heal in two main ways:

1. The aroma itself triggers the olfactory sense and acts on specific neurochemicals to achieve desired results.

2. The oils, when they contact tissue surfaces are absorbed, bind to fat cells, and then act on specific neurotransmitters.

3. Memories of smells are powerful. When a memory of an essential oil smell, combines with the effect it has on the body a person retains an impression of its ability to heal. For instance, if you use lavender oil before sleeping and it actually helps you fall asleep, the next time a person smells lavender oil they are likely to react.

Essential oils are very convenient, save time and are cost effective. Just by keeping the following short list on hand you can address multiple conditions. Starting an apothecary by purchasing a few essential oils is an easy way for you to start creating your home apothecary.

Please note: One cannot put essential oils directly on the skin. You have to dissolve them first in a substance.

Dissolve essentials oils in:

1. Hot water

   a. As a general rule, put three to five drops in a small pot for steaming. For a child one drop will be enough.

b. Twenty drops in a bathtub — remember to put the drops in the bath and swish them around thoroughly.

2. A carrier lotion or oil

   a. 3 drops per half teaspoon of oil is a general rule.

Steaming with Essential Oils

You can keep a ready supply of essential oils on hand for steaming if fresh herbs are not available.

There are 1,000 drops of essential oil in a 1-ounce vial. That is a compact form of healing and you can take these vials with you when you travel!

For steaming a good rule of thumb to follow is to use one drop for every 30 pounds you carry. If you weigh a hundred and thirty pounds, you will need about four drops.

When building your apothecary, keep one to two ounces of the following on hand:

3. **Peppermint** — Please read the Materia Medica on this herb. Using the essential oil is optional in cases where a person does not want to ingest peppermint. Mint is far too potent to use on the skin. Primarily you can steam with three drops of the oil under a steam tent as needed to open the sinus cavities. Mint is a very strong essential oil.

4. **Tea Tree** — is an excellent antibacterial oil that can be used on the skin (five drops to ½ teaspoon of carrier oil) for all types of bug bites, stings, and minor infections. Adjust the dose for children. One or two drops per ½ teaspoon is plenty.

5. **Lavender** — is a superior remedy for anxiety, and a sleep aid (five drops for ½ teaspoon of carrier oil) to heal minor wounds, burns, and insect bites. Apply to the back of the neck. Adjust the dose for children. One drop per ½ teaspoon is generally plenty for a child over the age of three or four depending on how much they weigh.

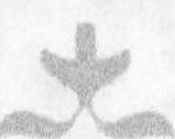

6. **Eucalyptus** — is a great remedy for steaming in case of cold, cough, or flu. It is an expectorant. Four drops for an adult in a small pot of steaming water is enough. This oil is OK for older children but probably too strong for younger children unless it is used in a diffuser specifically designed to permeate a room with an essence.

Sources

(1)   Gladstar, Rosemary, "The Art and Science of Herbalism", Chapters 1, 2 and 3, Vermont:Sage Mountain Press, 2014.

(2)   Hoffman, David, FNIMH, AHG, "The Complete Illustrated Holistic Herbal: A Safe and Practical Guide to Making and Using Herbal Remedies", Australia: Element Books Limited, 1996.

(3)   "Herbs for Healthy Aging: Natural Prescriptions for Vital Health" Vermont: Healing Arts Press, 2014.

(4)   Mojay, Gabriel, "Aromatherapy for Healing the Spirit: Restoring Emotional and Mental Balance with Essential Oils", Vermont: Healing Arts Press, 1997.

(5)   Tierra, Michael, L.Ac., OMD "The Way of Herbs", New York: Pocket Books 1998.

10 Guidelines for Using Remedies

At this point, you have become familiar with the Native American medicine chest. You have learned how to harness herbal power through preparing remedies in Chapter 9. Now we turn to the details of constructing your daily apothecary, stocking required herbs, and combining various remedies for everyday use:

- Chapter 10 will help you understand how much of what herbs to take when treating common ailments in different age groups

- Details on preparing these herbs are explained in the receipts in Chapter 12. This chapter shows the details of creating remedies.

- Complete your knowledge with Chapter 11, a bonus chapter and quick reference guide. Chapter 11 educates the reader on the multiple uses of one herb, and the similarities between many herbs.

To use your apothecary table effectively, familiarize yourself with the following principles to store your remedies and make them readily available:

1. Dosages for adults and children

2. The amount of herbs to keep on hand for the most basic situations

3. How to sequence the stages of a condition to know what herb to take at which stage

Everyone has the gift to heal. However, it requires skill and experience to treat yourself. Look carefully under the conditions in these guidelines to see what applies to the illness you are dealing with. Notice the stages of illness and the possibilities of healing each stage using different remedies. Be aware of conditions that may become too advanced for you to treat on your own. Seek help when needed from a qualified holistic practitioner.

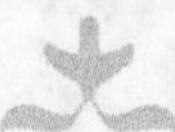

Please note: You can improve the taste of most teas with just a couple of pinches of either lemon zest, orange zest, or powdered mint. Honey is always an option.

Please review the following chapter regarding dosage carefully. You will have more clarity about the quantity of herbs needed for storage and, even more importantly, for consumption. Remember that you can usually buy common herbs by the ounce in your local health food store or co-op. Otherwise, you may harvest or grow them or purchase them in bulk online.

10.1 Learning About Herbal Dosages

Many of the herbs you gather will be mild. Therefore, the dosage of mild herbs may be higher, and the intake duration lengthened to make a difference in a long-term chronic condition. It is worth noting: master herbalists point out that ***most mistakes made when taking herbs occur due to taking the wrong dosage.*** Generally, the dose taken is too low, and so the person assumes that an herb is ineffective.

Commonly, people assume that they only need a pinch of herbs to make a difference, almost like the amount of spice you use to add flavor to a dish. But no, the human body is more complex than cooking a meal. When administering an herb this complexity must be taken into account even as a beginner. Please take the dosage instructions in this book seriously. Ask yourself the following questions if an herb does not work for you:

1. Would you be willing to take a larger dose if your herb is mild?

2. Do you need to have more patience with your healing process and wait for the herb to take effect?

3. Do you eat processed foods, foods out of season, or foods from other climates that slow your healing process down?

4. Is your healing process affected by any other lifestyle factors?

5. Do you need to see a practitioner for guidance? Encourage yourself to get the support you need.

Take some time to review the ancient practices and philosophy of Native Americans we talked about at the beginning of this book. It is sometimes challenging to fit this paradigm into a modern framework. However, basic suggestions like slowing down, reconnecting with family and community, spending time in nature, revisiting your priorities and seeking support are just as important as the herbal remedy itself. Perhaps, they are even more important.

You may see improvements from your remedy in just a few days. Remember that:

1. The standard herbal tea dose for a chronic condition is three cups a day.

2. The usual dose of an alcohol-based tincture is 1" or one dropper full three times daily.

3. The standard dosage of an herbal pill for chronic conditions is 500 mg to 1000 mg three times daily.

4. The usual dose for syrup is one teaspoon three times daily.

Simple conversion of mass units

Bulk herbs are generally sold by the ounce. Most herbal companies require a minimum purchase of 4 ounces. Conversions from ounces to tablespoons and teaspoons follow.

Common Measurement Conversions for Herbal Substances

1 ounce = 2 tablespoons and 6 teaspoons

2 ounces = 4 tablespoons and 12 teaspoons

4 ounces = 8 tablespoons and 24 teaspoons

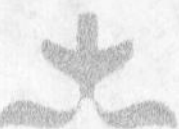

10.2 Self Monitoring and when to Seek Medical Support

Learn the baselines first. Check-in with yourself daily. Do you notice any changes? Three times daily means morning, afternoon, and evening. Carry your tincture, tea, pills, or syrup in your purse or backpack so that you will not miss a dose when you leave the house.

Last but not least — drink plenty of water! Herbs act on particular systems and often release toxins from them. Astringent herbs literally squeeze liquid from the cells to release excesses and allow room for cells to renew. It takes extra water to facilitate all of the jobs that herbs perform.

1. Do you feel dehydrated after taking your herbs?

2. Do you feel a headache after taking your herb?

3. Do you feel nausea after taking your herb?

If any of these feelings apply to you, try drinking more water. If that does not help, call a practitioner.

10.3 Remedies fo Kids

If not indicated differently, kids can take the same remedies as adults but with different dosages. To determine the right dosage for children, let's look at Cowling's rule. It is a formula to calculate a dose of herbs for children. Getting children to taste medicine is not always easy. You have to be creative. Sometimes children (or adults for that matter) take medicine more easily in yogurt, applesauce, or pudding. Do whatever works for the individual.

Cowling's Rule is the year of the child's next birthday divided by 24. So if your child turns four next year and you divide four by 24 you will administer *1/6* of the adult dosage. [5]

Children often like tea. It is comforting and warm and especially if you put a little honey in it, they usually drink it. An adult tea dosage is one cup. For a child give the following amount of tea:

1. Children 1 year or less — two teaspoons

2. Children 2 to 4 years — three teaspoons

3. Children 4 to 7 years — 1 tablespoon

4. Children 7 to 11 years — 2 tablespoons

10.4 Your Basic Herbal First Aid Kit

(Pain, Inflammation, Burns, Cuts, Bleeding, Toothache, Immunity)

Pain and Inflammation

Your first line of defense for pain and inflammation is **White Willow Bark**. Take 500 mg three times daily. Combine this with the **Devil's Club Salve or the Devil's Club tea** for more severe chronic pain. The next level would be acute pain, for instance, from an injury or surgery. Then instead of Devil's Club salve or tea, use **Arnica Oil** every three to four hours.

*   **White Willow Bark Tea or capsules**
    Keep 4 oz of White Willow Bark powder/ or pills 120 caps 500 mg on hand.
    For all types of pain, internal and external.

*   **Devil's Club Tea and Salve**
    Keep 4 oz Devil's Club bark or bark powder on hand.

---

[5]   Gladstar, Rosemary, "Art and Science of Herbalism", Chapter 4, p.7

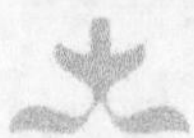

Use the tea or salve for chronic to acute pain or inflammation. Devil's Club is more potent than White Willow Bark.

- **Arnica Oil**
  Keep 4oz of Arnica aerial parts and 4 oz olive oil on hand.
  Use for acute or sudden pain, bruises, swelling, and inflammation. Not for cuts or on skin that is not intact. Please follow the recipe to make this remedy in chapter 12. You will need 4 oz of Arnica aerial parts to create the Oil.

Burns and cuts

Minor burns and cuts need immediate attention. Keep plantain on hand so you can make a poultice if required.

- **Plantain leaf poultice**
  Keep 6 oz of cut leaves on hand.
  Makes a poultice for burns or cuts.

Stop Bleeding

If you get a cut in the kitchen or while minor gardening, making a **Yarrow** poultice will stop the bleeding. After the bleeding has stopped, ultimately, you can make a **Plantain** poultice to heal the skin.

- **Yarrow leaf poultice**
  Keep 4oz of yarrow leaves on hand.
  Subdues fever or makes a poultice to stop bleeding.

Toothache

- **Sage leaf tea**
  Keep 4 oz — 8 oz Sage leaf on hand.
  It is beneficial to have a decent amount of Sage on hand. One of them is to stop a toothache. Make a cup of **Sage** tea. Keep it in a jar in the refrigerator and swish with a tablespoon of the tea in your mouth four times daily.

Fever

- **Yarrow leaf tea**
  Keep 4 oz on hand.
  Subdues fever or stops bleeding when you apply a poultice.

Cold or Sinus Infection

- **Peppermint Essential Oil Steam**
  Keep a 1 oz bottle on hand for steaming.

Cough

- **Eucalyptus Essential Oil Steam**
  Keep a 1 oz bottle on hand.
  Use for steaming to reduce coughing and mucus. Steam alongside the antiviral tincture and the Elderberry syrup.

- **Elderberry Syrup**
  Keep a 16 oz bottle on hand.
  Boosts immunity and shortens the duration of cold, cough, and flu.

Flu

- **Elderberry Syrup**
  Keep one 16 oz bottle on hand.
  You will need to keep one cup of dried elderberries, one cup of honey, one cinnamon stick, one inch of fresh Ginger, and three clove buds on hand to make this recipe.
  Review the recipe for the ingredients and make one batch of syrup every season. Boosts immunity and shortens illness duration.

- **Peppermint Essential Oil Steam**
  Keep 1 oz on hand.
  It opens the lungs and helps clear congestion.

- **Antiviral tincture**
  Keep four two-ounce bottles on hand.

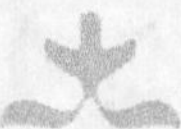

They will last six months to a year, depending on your family size. See Chapter 12 for the exact amounts of herbal substances needed; the list is lengthy. The antiviral tincture clears chest congestion reduces fever and body aches. Use the tincture at the chronic dose level if you feel a cough developing suddenly.

Combination Cold, Cough, Flu

- **Peppermint Oil Steam**
  Keep a 1 oz bottle on hand for the whole family.
  Start steaming three times daily with **only one drop when the sniffles begin. Peppermint is powerful and can cause a burn if you get too close to the steam.**

- **Mullein (or Yarrow)**
  Keep 4 oz of either herb, or both, on hand.
  Yarrow and Mullein have similar qualities and are the same strength. Make the tea for a child at the first sign of a cough. It is safe for a child to take Mullein tea and Elderberry syrup. Even if a child does not have the flu, the Elderberry will boost immunity and shorten the duration of the cough.

- **Elderberry Syrup**
  Keep 16 oz on hand each season for a family of four.
  The syrup will be your first line of defense for cold, cough, and flu. It is probably one of the top three most important things to have on hand. It only lasts about eight weeks if refrigerated.

If the cold or cough worsens, consider adding a **Yarrow Poultice** to the chest.

One may give **Yarrow tea** to reduce the fever.

Stomach Ache

- **Chamomile flowers tea**
  Keep 4 oz of Chamomile aerial parts on hand to calm the stomach ache of a child or adult.

Ear Ache

- **Mullein ear oil**
  Keep 1 oz of the oil on hand.
  You will only need 2 oz of dried Mullein flowers to make the ear oil. So, keep 2 oz of dried Mullein flowers on hand. The oil will last for two years if kept in the dark.

Headache

- **Lemon Balm tea**
  Keep 4 oz of dried aerial parts on hand

10.5 Immunity

We all need to pay careful attention to boosting immunity whenever possible. The very best remedy is prevention itself! It is vital to consume substances regularly that boost our immunity to have reserves for unforeseen circumstances.

Generally speaking, one ounce of an herb will last a child a week. Three to four ounces a week of most herbs is suitable for an adult.

Take one of the following depending on what is best for you and your family. You can combine the cookies or lozenges with any tea for daily support — just pay attention to the different dosage requirements for adults and children.

- **Rose Hips tea**
  Keep 4 oz on hand.

- **Pine Needle tea**
  Keep 1 cup of dried needles on hand.
  Take the tea daily as needed. Feel free to switch your daily immune-boosting formula. You do not have to take the same one all the time.

- **Echinacea Tea**
  Keep 8 oz of Echinacea leaves on hand.

Take the tea daily for up to three months.

- **Echinacea/Ginger/Lemon Tonic**
(Prepare two quarts weekly)
Keep on hand 4 oz of Echinacea, three inches of Ginger, 1 lemon and honey to taste.

- Varieties of **edible mushrooms 1 lb per week** for two adults
You will have to see if your children will eat mushrooms. If they do — fabulous! One tablespoon a couple of times a week for a child should be fine.

- **Throat Lozenges made with Echinacea Powder**
Good to have a batch on hand. The cookies last for a couple of weeks if stored in an airtight container. One a day for prevention is enough.

- **Immune-boosting cookies**
Good to have a batch on hand. The cookies last for a couple of weeks if stored in an airtight container. One a day for prevention is enough.

- **Elderberry syrup**
Keep 16 oz on hand for two adults and two children.
Elderberry syrup can be combined with any tea, plus the throat lozenges or cookies as a sort of wellness package.

Please note: Onions and garlic are excellent immune boosters. Cook with them whenever possible. Both onions and garlic are blood pressure and blood sugar-stabilizing foods.

10.6 Recovering from illness

- **Oatstraw Tea**
Keep 8 oz on hand.
It is an essential herb to keep all year long for fatigue, weakness, and exhaustion. Take the tea as needed for long-term support.

10.7 Worms and Parasites

- **Mugwort tincture**
  Keep 4 oz Mugwort aerial parts on hand (along with 8 oz of the alcohol of your choice to make the tincture)
  Mugwort is a strong herb. The dosage will depend on how severe the condition is. Try the chronic dose and then increase it to four times a day if needed.
  Make four two-ounce tincture bottles to last a small family for up to two years. However, the tincture will store for several years.

10.8 Anxiety, Lethargy & Concentration

Anxiety

- **Chamomile tea**
  Keep 4 oz of dried flowers on hand for purposes mentioned so far, or anxiety.

- **Lemon Balm tea**
  Keep 4 oz of dried flowers on hand for purposes mentioned so far, or anxiety.

Lethargy and lack of concentration

- **Peppermint Essential Oil Steam**
  Keep 1 oz on hand for steaming.
  Again, remember to steam with one drop only and keep the face at least a foot above the steam while you close your eyes.

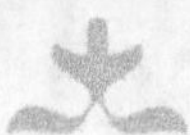

10.9 Middle Aged to Senior Phase of Life Remedies

Immunity

Please review the Immunity section.

Chronic Pain

Please review the Chronic Pain section.

Cold, Cough, and Flu

Please review the Cold, Cough, and Flu section.

Memory Issues

- **Rosemary Hair Oil**
  Keep 4 oz of the oil extraction on hand. To make the extraction you will need 4 oz of the leaves and 4 oz of olive oil. Apply one to two times daily to the scalp and massage the oil into your head thoroughly.

Anemia

- **Nettle/Red Clover Tea**
  Keep 4 oz on hand.

- **Red Clover**
  Keep 4 oz on hand.
  You will combine equal parts to make the Nettle/Red Clover tea. You can take this long term safely. It is also an excellent nutritional and immune-boosting tonic.

Kidney Stone Prevention and Urinary Tract Infection

- **Horsetail Uva Ursi Tea**
  Keep 4 oz of Horsetail aerial parts and 4 oz of Uva Ursi on hand.

  Combine equal parts of these herbs to make this tea for two weeks. Then take a break for one week and resume if problems persist. Additionally, for urinary tract infections, you can take ¼ cup of cranberry juice three times daily to clean the walls of the urinary system.

Hypertension and Blood Sugar Stabilization

- **Ginger Root tea**
  Keep a small cluster, or several inches of Ginger root on hand. Take three cups of tea daily for mild hypertension and blood sugar control. You can have either one condition or the other, or both. Ginger is an excellent way to address either issue, plus it will detoxify the blood and aid digestion. Ginger is a perfect remedy for aging in general.

Energy and Concentration

The following remedies are arranged from the least strong to the strongest. Start with the first and move down the list progressively. However, do not take all the remedies at the same time! It will be too stimulating.

If you have gathered your herbs as directed up to this point, you will have the supplies needed for the following remedies.

1. Peppermint Steam three times daily

   or

2. Echinacea/Ginger/Lemon Tonic, take three cups daily.
   Refer to the recipe for the portions. you will need to make a few quarts per week so plan accordingly.

   or

3. Ginseng tea — Take two cups daily, in the morning and after-
    noon.

    Keep 4 oz of dried American Ginseng root on hand.

Alternatively, you can make a vegetable soup and add *one ounce of Ginseng* to the soup as you boil it. Ensure that the Ginseng root is simmering in the soup for ½ hour. One or two bowls a day is a mild remedy that the whole family can consume.

Consuming the soup and steaming with mint oil are fine to do at separate times of the day. Both are gentle remedies and work well together.

Weight Loss

These weight loss remedies are meant to address congestion in the liver, break up fat cells, flush them out of the system, and tone the tissues to extract toxins.

- **Lemon/Ginger Echinacea Tonic**
  Keep a small cluster of Ginger, five lemons, and 4 oz Echinacea on hand. It will last you several days if you make a quart per day.
  For weight loss, take 3 cups daily. It is a wonderful immune-boosting remedy and very warming for those who get cold quickly.

Or you can take:

- **Nettle/Rose Hips Tea**
  Keep 4 oz of Nettle and 4 oz of Rose Hips on hand.
  The tea will last you about two weeks if you take three cups daily. Nettle/Rose Hips tea is highly nutritious and also immune-boosting. It is a reliable remedy for both weight loss and daily immunity and a bit stronger than the tonic above. Take three cups daily. It is not as warming as the Echinacea/Lemon/Ginger tonic due to the absence of Ginger.

Anxiety, Insomnia, and Depression

Anxiety is often the cause of insomnia. First, consider your anxiety level. Sometimes it is hard to understand how much anxiety is present. Mild herbs for anxiety include **Lemon Balm** and **Chamomile**. If you have some routine anxiety, three cups per day of either tea should be enough. If you have chronic issues with anxiety, then **Hops** or **California Poppy** tea may be more effective.

Most of the suggestions for insomnia will apply to anxiety as well. However, just take one tea at a time, unless you use Oatstraw tea along with one of the other herbs in this section.

For **insomnia**, you may want to start your tea consumption later in the morning so that your last dose of tea is an hour before you go to sleep. Sedatives relax the nervous system while nervines tone the nervous system. Hops and California Poppy contain both actions.

- **Hops tea**
  Keep 4 oz on hand.
  Take three cups of tea daily. It is milder than California poppy. If you need something more robust for a particularly disturbed sleep cycle, take the California Poppy.

- **California Poppy Flowers tea**
  Keep 4 oz on hand.
  Take two to three cups of tea daily. It is a strong sedative and will work for both anxiety and insomnia.

If you have problems with pain at night that keep you awake, consider taking **White Willow Bark 1000 to 1500 mg** one-half hour before sleep. White Willow Bark relieves pain and is a sedative. However, it is not a very strong sedative, so you may want to combine it with either the Hops or the California Poppy for pain.

- **Rose Massage Oil**
  Keep 4 oz of the extracted oil on hand. To make it you will need 4 oz of dried rose petals and 6 oz of olive oil.

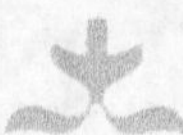

Rose oil is beneficial to keep on hand for all family members. It will help a child relax before bed if you give them a light back massage.

If sleep is very problematic for adults, self-massage or a professional massage with your **Rose massage oil** may help.

A problematic sleep cycle takes time to adjust. You cannot just 'catch up' on missed sleep all at once. Please be patient with yourself while you restore and your hormonal cycle changes. It can take several weeks and sometimes several months.

For restoration, there is hardly a better herb than Oatstraw. Oatstraw tea is something that is taken long-term. It has a more stable shelf life than flowers and even some herbal leaves.

- **Oatstraw**
  Keep 8 oz, a good supply of this herb on hand.
  Oatstraw is a user-friendly herb for everyone in the family. At some point during the year, almost everyone is likely to suffer from exhaustion. Within three days of taking this tea, most people will notice a difference. It is a subtle herb. It reaches the adrenals, soothes, and restores. One of the main benefits of Oatstraw is that it complements any herb. It has a gentle, supportive action that enhances the actions of other herbs. This book is not about the more complex actions of herbal formulation. However, it is worth learning about all this herb can do in further herbal studies.

- **Saw Palmetto**
  Keep sixty 500 mg capsules on hand.
  Saw Palmetto is a wonderful therapeutic herb for those in the prime of their life, raising children, forging ahead in careers, and suffering from fatigue. It has a unique action of restoring the reproductive/genital system. This herb is worth taking if fatigue affects sexual function, especially men.
  Keep the capsules on hand. They will last up to two years.

10.10 Beauty

Beauty and wellness depend on proper nutrition, adequate sleep, healthy family life, social connections, and other aspects. However, herbs can certainly help, and it is worth making your beauty products with ingredients that you can trust.

This book presents a weekly nighttime regime:

1. Steam the pores open with the **Rose** petal face steam.

2. Apply the **Nettle Green Clay** face mask after patting the face dry from steaming.

3. Ending with a thin application of the **Rose** massage oil.

Repeat once weekly. The routine pampers and restores.

For the above practice, you need:

- **Rose Petals**
  Keep 6 oz on hand.
  You will use this to make the Rose massage oil and also for the Rose petal/Sage face steam.

- **Sage, 2oz**
- **Nettle**
  Keep 2 oz on hand
  (in addition to what you have already gathered from these guidelines)

- **Green Clay**
  Keep 2 oz on hand.

10.11 Sexual and Reproductive Health

At this point in your herbal shopping, you will have acquired all of the herbs needed for this section.

Sexual health improves through lifestyle factors, especially sleep. The second factor to address is underlying issues such as anxiety and de-

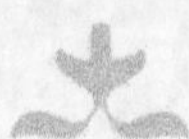

pression. Another factor that increases sexual vitality and confidence in weight loss. Think carefully about whether any of these issues apply to you. When reviewing the following section, choose the most appropriate tea for you. Four ounces of the ingredient you choose will be enough for the standard dose while consuming the tea for two weeks.

The remedies proceed from number one to number four by order of strength. Review the formulas for anxiety, depression, and insomnia very carefully. If you decide to make these formulas, go back and look at the Materia Medica. If you are uncertain what you need, follow the guidance of a practitioner.

Anxiety and Depression

- **Lemon Balm tea, Chamomile tea** are mild remedies for anxiety. **Keep 4 oz of either herb on hand.**

- **Hops tea or California Poppy tea**
  Either herb is a mild to medium strength remedy for anxiety. **Keep 4 oz of either herb on hand.**

- **Rose Massage oil and Rose tea** will help depression. **Keep 4 oz of the extracted oil on hand.**

- **Mint tea** is a mild stimulant for depression and can provide temporary relief.
  Keep 4 oz of Peppermint or Spearmint leaves on hand.
  Most Mint leaves have very similar qualities.

Fatigue

Review the Insomnia section above and follow those guidelines.

Sexual vitality

Try the Ginseng tea above first, two cups daily, taken before 3:00 pm. You could combine this with the Rose Massage oil.

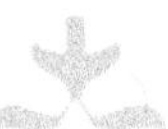

Sexual Vitality and Reproductive Health

Ginseng/Hops/Oatstraw/ Dried Blackberry Tincture (for erectile dysfunction, strength, endurance)

Review the recipe for your supplies and keep **two two-ounce dropper bottles** on hand.

This formula is for invigoration and combatting long-term fatigue.

Substitute Saw Palmetto for Ginseng during the preparation if you have experienced reproductive issues. See the recipe for Saw Palmetto/ Hops/Oatstraw/ Dried Blackberry Tincture (for reproductive health, strength, and endurance) for your supply list.

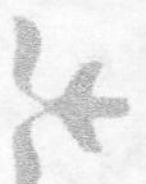

11 Overview List of Conditions and Corresponding Healing Herbs

The following table provides a list of herbal uses at a glance for quick reference. Notice that you can sometimes substitute one herb for another. It is also interesting to note how many times the "super herbs" or "adaptogens" show up as possible remedies for multiple conditions.

ailment	symptom	Herbal aids							
Abdominal Cramping		Black Cohosh	Chamomile	Meadowsweet	Sage				
Exhaustion		Oatstraw	Pine	Sage					
Aging	skin	Rose	Plantain						
	hair	Rosemary	Nettles						
Allergies		Goldenrod	Oak Buds	Nettles					
Anemia		Dock	Greenbrier	Red Clover	Nettles				
Ankles, swollen		Arnica	Echinacea	Rose Hips	Devil's Club				

Anxiety		Chamomile	Lemon Balm	Oat Seed	Sage			
Arterial Plaque		Ginger	Echinacea					
Arthritis		Arnica	Devil's Club	Ginger	Meadowsweet	Pine	White Willow	
Asthma		Goldenrod	Nettle					
Bladder Infection		Uva Ursi	Rose Hips	Saw Palmetto				
Blood Pressure	high	Ginger						
	low	Rosemary						
	cardiotonic	Milkweed						
Bones	aching	Boneset	Devil's Club					
	injured	Arnica	Devil's Club					
Bowels	distention of	Ginger						
	infection of	Ginger						
	movement of		Chamomile	Devil's Club				
	putrification of		Ginger					
Bronchial	congestion		Boneset	Milkweed	Ginger	Mullein		
	dry cough	Elderberry	Ginger	Sage				

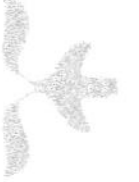

	wet cough	Black Cohosh	Ginger	Milkweed	Sage	Mullein			
	cold chest		Ginger	Milkweed					
	hot chest			Mint					
Cholesterol		Ginger							
Circulation		Ginger	Rosemary	Yarrow					
Constipation		Cattails	Devil's Club	Ginger					
Depression		Oatstraw	Rosemary	Rose					
Diabetes		Ginger							
Diarrhea		Blackberry	Black Gum Bark	Sage					
Diaper Rash		Cattails	Mullein leaf	Plantain					
Earache		Mullein							
Emotional Challenges		California Poppy	Chamomile	Dandelion flr.	Lemon Balm	Oatstraw	Sage	Rose	Rosemary
Fatigue		Blackberries	Devils' Club	Mushrooms	Oatstraw	Rosemary	Sage		
Flu (antiviral)		Elderberry	Boneset	Devil's Club	Ginger				
Fever		Black Gum Bark	Boneset	Devil's Club	Elderberry	Meadowseet	White Willow	Yarrow	
Fungus		Devils' Club	Mugwort						
Headaches		Lemon Balm	Mint	While Willow	Sage				

Hemorrhoids		Blackberry Leaf	Plantain						
Hypoglycemia		Ginger	Ginseng						
Immune boost		Elderberry	Ginger	Ginseng	Mushrooms	Pine Needles	Rose Hips		
Indigestion		Chamomile	Lemon Balm	Mint	Sage				
Inflammation		Chamomile	Dandelion	Devils' Club	Ginger	Goldenrod	Lemon Balm	Meadowsweet	Oak
		Pine	Saw Palmetto	White Willow	Yerba Santa				
Insomnia		California Poppy	Chamomile	Lemon Balm	Hops				
Kidney	infection	Uva Ursi	Milkweed						
	adrenal fatigue	Blackberries	Ginseng	Mushrooms	Pine	Rose Hips			
Lethargy		Devils' Club	Ginseng	Mint	Mushrooms	Oak(Acorns)	Oat Seed	Rosemary	Sage
Liver	congestion	Black Cohosh	Dandelion	Dock	Echinacea	Ginger	Greenbrier	Mint	Nettles
		Yerba Santa							
Lung	congestion		Boneset	Ginger	Milkweed	Mullein	Yerba Santa		
	inflammation		Boneset	Mullein	Yerba Santa				
	infection		Boneset	Ginger	Mullein				
Memory Loss		Rosemary	Mushrooms						

Menstruation	regulation	Black Cohosh	Saw Palmetto					
	hot flashes	Sage	Black Cohosh					
	night sweats	Sage	Nettles	Rose Hips				
	weight gain	Echinacea	Lemon Balm	Oatstraw				
	depression	Mint	Hops	Rosemary				
	insomnia	California Poppy	Chamomile					
Muscular	soreness	Arnica	Chamomile	Black Cohosh	Devil's Club	Meadowsweet	Rosemary	
	spasms	Black Cohosh	Boneset	Devil's Club	White Willow			
	strain	Arnica	Dandelion	Devil's Club				
	inflammation	Arnica	Devil's Club	Ginger	Nettles	Meadowsweet		
Nausea		Ginger						
Parasites		Black Gum Bark	Mugwort					
Poison Ivy		Cattail	Greenbrier	Plantain				
Prostate Issues		Saw Palmetto	Uva Ursi					
Rheumatism		Arnica	Meadowsweet	Nettles	Rheumatism			
Sinus Infections		Mint						
Sexual Health		Ginseng	Rose	Saw Palmetto				

Stings		Cattail	Plantain					
Throat (sore)		Elderberry	Ginger	Lemon Balm	Mint	Mullein	Pine	Rose Hips
Tooth Pain		Oak Bark	Sage					
Vaginitis		Oak Bark	Black Gum Bark	Saw Palmetto				
Varicose Veins		Ginger	Dock	Red Clover	Yarrow			
Vomiting	to stop	Mint	Black Gum Bark					
	to induce	Greenbrier						
Weight Loss		Echinacea	Ginger	Nettles				
Worms		Black Gum Bark	Mugwort					
Wounds		Cattail	Plantain	Yarrow	Greenbrier	Milkweed		

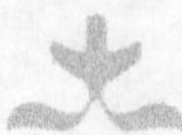

12 Herbal dispensatory — Remedies and Recipes for different needs

12.1 Remedies for Cold, Cough, and Flu

Elderberry Syrup
For cold, cough, and flu

One cup of dried elderberries
One tablespoon grated ginger
Three whole cloves
One cinnamon stick
1/2 teaspoon of orange zest
Three cups of boiling water
¾ cup of honey

In a medium-sized saucepan, heat the water until it boils. Add the elderberries and turn the heat down to simmer. Add the ginger, cloves, cinnamon stick, and orange zest. Continue to simmer and reduce the syrup by half.

Strain into a bowl or measuring cup.
(Discard the berries or boil them again in three cups of water to make tea!)
Add the honey at the end and stir well.
Put the mixture into a glass jar and label it. Elderberry syrup lasts up to eight weeks in the refrigerator.

Take one teaspoon every three hours in case of flu. Take one teaspoon three times a day for a cold or cough.

Mullein Ear Oil (safe for children)
for ear infections

1. Simmer two teaspoons of mullein flowers in ¼ cup olive oil for 20 minutes.

2. Strain into a glass vessel, then pour into a dropper bottle.

3. Let it cool.

4. Put one drop into the ear canal gently and massage the bony bump behind the ear to allow the oil to settle.

5. Lay on the opposite side and put in the second drop. Massage the back of that ear for a minute or so.

6. Two drops, three times daily, especially before bed, will help clear an ear infection.

Lung/Sinus Clearing Steam (Mint)

Prepare a mint tea infusion per standard infusion directions with a quart of boiling water and one tablespoon of either dried or fresh herb. Let the herbs sit and steam in a small pot with the burner turned off. Cover your head with a hand towel to make a tent. Standing over the pot, breathe in the steam deeply until the vapors fade. Cover up with warm clothing afterward.

White Willow Bark Tea
for pain, inflammation, and insomnia

Take this tea for pain inflammation and before bed to ensure a pain-free night of sleep. (If you would rather purchase the capsules, take 500mg twice daily and one last dose of 1500 mg before sleeping. After a couple of weeks using this routine, discontinue the herbs for a few days, then resume if pain continues.)

Boil one quart of water.

1. Add a tablespoon of white willow bark.

2. Decoct the herbs for 20 minutes.

3. Strain them into a clean glass vessel.

4. Drink three cups, morning, afternoon, and evening.

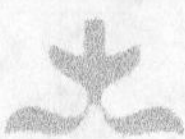

Most teas store for three to four days.

Yerba Buena Cough Syrup (Pine, Yerba Buena)
For cold, cough, and flu

Three ounces Yerba Buena dried aerial parts
¼ cup chopped pine needles
One tablespoon grated ginger
1/2 teaspoon of lemon zest
One tablespoon mint
Four cups of boiling water
¾ cup of honey

In a medium-sized saucepan, heat the water until it boils. Add the Yerba Buena and pine and turn the heat down to simmer. Add the ginger, lemon zest, and mint. Continue to simmer until the mixture is reduced by half.

Strain into a bowl or measuring cup. Discard the herbs.
Add the honey at the end and stir well.
Put the mixture into a glass jar and label it. This syrup will last up to eight weeks in the refrigerator.

Take one teaspoon every three hours in case of acute cough. Take one teaspoon three times a day or, as needed, for a mild cough.

Antiviral Tincture (Boneset/Butterfly Weed/Meadowsweet/Lemon Balm)

This recipe is a little more complex than a simpling recipe using one herb, but the same principle applies. You will combine the herbs and then cover them completely with alcohol.

Combine:
3 ounces Boneset (reduce fever, body ache, and coughing)
3 ounces Butterfly Weed Root (expectorant, reduces fever, dispels toxins)
2 ounces Yarrow (expectorant, reduces fever, anti-inflammatory)
1-ounce Ginseng Root) 2 ounces (immunostimulant, increases stamina)
2 ounces Oatstraw (demulcent, soothes tissues)

Place ingredients in a glass jar. Cover with alcohol and let sit in a cool dark place for 21 days—strain and store in a glass jar. You can also put your tincture into 2-ounce dropper bottles.

If you get the flu, which is an acute condition, at the onset of symptoms, you will need to begin taking this tincture 1" at least every four hours. As symptoms persist or even increase, take this tincture 1" every three hours. Decrease the dose gradually as symptoms decrease.

Keep taking the chronic dose, 1" three times daily for a week even after symptoms subside. Viruses have a way of embedding themselves deep inside the tissues. Viruses like to hide. Taking this tincture for an additional week ensures that the deeper levels of the illness subside.

Throat Lozenges (Ginger, Sage)

You will be surprised how simple it is to prepare your throat lozenges.

1. Prepare one ounce of Tragacanth (a natural gum you can order online) by melting it in 1 pint of boiling water.

2. After melting, soak the mixture for twenty-four hours.

3. The following day, beat the mixture to make it smooth.

4. Strain it through two layers of cheesecloth to make a sticky liquid.

5. Add one tablespoon of brown sugar to the liquid.

6. Add equal parts ginger powder and sage powder until the mixture thickens into a paste. You will probably need a heaping tablespoon of each herbal powder.

7. Put cornflour on a surface to roll out the paste.

8. Roll out the paste covering it with the cornflour.

9. Let it cool, and then cut it into small bite-sized squares.

10. Store the lozenges in a tin or glass container.

Take the lozenges as needed.

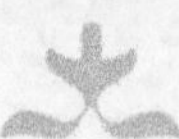

Echinacea/Ginger/Lemon First Aid Tonic
for increasing immunity

1. Prepare one tablespoon of grated Ginger

2. Measure 1 tablespoon of Echinacea

3. Cut one lemon into quarters

4. Set aside ¼ cup of honey

Decoct the ginger root in a quart of boiling water for twenty minutes.
Add the echinacea and let it infuse for another 15 minutes.
Strain the mixture into a bowl.
Add the juice of one lemon.
Add ¼ cup of honey (or sweeten to your taste)

Store in a glass container in the refrigerator for up to five days.

Immune Boosting Cookies for Children

Mixing powdered herbs into a cookie is a great way to distribute tasty
preventative medicine or heal an already ill child.

1. Grind the dried fruits of your choice in a food processor or
    grinder

2. Stir in coconut.

3. Mix in some peanut butter or another nut butter until you can
    roll the cookies into balls.

4. Measure how many cookies your batch will make.

5. Measure the amount of powdered herb your child will need in
    one cookie using the dosage measurements provided.

6. Measure the herb powder and mix it into the cookie dough.

7. Roll the cookies and serve.

Herbal powder options include Echinacea, Nettle, Yarrow, Mullein,
or Mint. One or two cookies a day, in addition to tea dosages, makes
healing more fun.

12.2 Remedies for Skin, Hair, Muscular Pain, Stomach and Headache, Allergies and Memory

The following recipes are for oil extractions. Flowers and leaves are extracted and stored without cooking. Roots and heavier mediums are slow-cooked overnight.

Plantain Oil Extraction
For mild skin issues and itching

1. In a quart-sized jar, place 1 cup of your dried plantain or two cups of fresh plantain.

2. Cover the herb entirely with whatever oil you choose (Olive, almond, avocado, apricot are good choices.)

3. Cover the jar with a lid.

4. Store in a cool, dark place for thirty to forty days. It takes a long time for oil extractions to complete.

5. Shake the jar a couple of times a week to mix your ingredients.

6. After the extraction is finished, strain the oil into a strainer lined with cheesecloth that sits over a bowl.

7. After the oil drips through the cloth, gather the edges of the cloth. Twist and squeeze all of the oil out into the bowl.

8. Pour the finished extraction into a glass jar.

9. Store in a cool, dark place. Oleolites have a fair degree of shelf stability and will last for a couple of years when stored properly.

Plantain Poultice
for Wounds, Burns, and Skin issues

A Plantain poultice is a very powerful healer of skin tissue, and extracts toxins and infections from the skin. It has the power to reach beneath the subdermal layers. The herb is remarkable!

1. Gather ½ cup of dried leaves or 1 cup of fresh leaves.

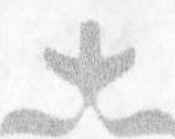

2. Macerate them with ¼ cup water. Add more if needed to make a paste.

3. Spread the paste on the affected area

4. Cover with a 12" by 12 " clean cotton cloth (a sturdy paper towel is also fine)

5. Let the poultice work for 20 minutes to a half hour.

You can reuse this twice. then make a fresh batch. Repeat the process two to three times daily.

Devil's Club Oil Extraction
for Pain and Inflammation
(Please see the video referenced below for complete uses of this herb by a native practitioner.) [6]

1. One cup of Devil's Club

2. One and a half cups of olive oil to cover the chopped dried Devil's Club

Place the oil and dried root in a quart-sized glass jar. Sink the pot into three inches of water in a crockpot. Cover the crockpot and let the mixture cook slowly overnight.

In the morning, cool, and then strain your oil into a clean glass jar. Store in a cool, dark, dry place. It makes an excellent massage oil to rub on sore and painful areas. Do not use it on broken skin.

Devil's Club Salve
for Pain and Inflammation

1. Warm 1 cup of Devil's Club oil that you have finished extracting in a double boiler.

2. Add ¼ cup of beeswax and stir until melted.

3. Pour into small jars or metal tins — cap and store in a cool, dark place.

---

6   Watkins, Helen, "Devil's Club" Traditional Uses by the Tlingit Native American tribal elders of Alaska, April 1, 2016, Seen on: *https://www.youtube.com/watch?v=DyUssKc2T-LQ, January 22, 2022.*

4. Apply as needed for pain and inflammation.

Please note that both the oil and the salve produce the same result. Salves are fun to make and easy to store. They also make great gifts. So it's up to you whether you want to use the Devil's Club oil or the salve.

Arnica Oil Extraction
for Pain Bruising and Inflammation

1. In a quart-sized jar, place 1 cup of your dried herb or two cups of a fresh herb.

2. Cover the herb entirely with whatever oil you choose (olive, almond, avocado, apricot are good choices)

3. Cover the jar with a lid.

4. Store in a cool, dark place for thirty to forty days. It takes a long time for oil extractions to complete.

5. Shake the jar a couple of times a week to mix your ingredients.

6. After the extraction is finished, pour the oil into a strainer lined with cheesecloth that sits over a bowl.

7. After the oil drips through the cloth, gather the edges of the cloth. Twist and squeeze all of the oil into the bowl, utilising the last drop of your extraction.

8. Pour the finished extraction into a glass jar.

9. Store in a cool, dark place. Oleolites have a fair degree of shelf stability and will last for a couple of years when stored properly.

Rosemary Hair Oil
for Memory, Energy, *and* Beautiful Hair

1. One cup of olive oil

2. One cup dried Rosemary leaves or 1 ½ fresh Rosemary leaves.

Place the oil in a quart-sized glass jar. Sink the pot into three inches of water in a crockpot. Cover the crockpot and let the mixture cook overnight.

Cool, and then strain in the morning into a clean glass jar. Store in a cool, dark, dry place. Take about a nickel-sized amount of the oil and rub it on your palms. Thoroughly massage it into your scalp. It increases circulation to the scalp and restores both memory, stimulants cognition, and fortifies hair as well.

Devil's Club Tea
for Inflammation

1. Boil one quart of water.

2. Add one tablespoon of Devil's Club bark..

3. Decoct for 20 minutes.

4. Strain into a clean glass vessel.

5. Drink three cups, morning, afternoon, and evening.

Most teas store for three to four days. You can use the Devil's Club oil externally along with the tea twice daily if you have a higher level of pain in a particular area.

Hops Tea
for insomnia

If you are having trouble sleeping, Hops, a medium-level nervine and sedative, can help you release the worries of the day.

1. Boil one quart of water.

2. Add three teaspoons of dried Hops aerial parts.

3. Infuse for 15 minutes.

4. Strain into a clean glass vessel

5. Drink three cups, morning, afternoon, and evening.

Most teas store for three to four days. If insomnia is an ongoing issue, taking an herbal sleep tea like Hops for a couple of weeks to catch up on missed sleep is fine. Alternatively you can use other milder herbs instead, like Sage, Chamomile and Lemon Balm.

Ginseng Tea
for stamina and to increase libido

1. Boil one quart of water.

2. Add one tablespoon of Ginseng root.

3. Decoct the root for 20 minutes.

4. Strain the decoction into a clean glass vessel.

5. Drink only two cups, morning and afternoon. Ginseng is too stimulating to take in the late afternoon and evening.

Most teas store for three to four days. Ginseng tea will increase both stamina and libido. Alternatively, you can decoct two tablespoons of the root, tied in cheesecloth in a typical vegetable soup. A milder dose of Ginseng along with vegetables and broth is excellent preventative medicine for the whole family!

**Chamomile Tea — Children and Adults
for digestive distress**

Take this tea for depression or mild relaxation. Chamomile tea is also used for mild colds and sore throats.

1. Boil one quart of water.

2. Add 1 heaping tablespoon of dried Chamomile.

3. Infuse the herbs for 15 minutes.

4. Strain them into a clean glass vessel

5. Drink three cups, morning, afternoon, and evening.

Most teas store for three to four days.

Anti-Allergen Tea with Nettle and Goldenrod

Take this tea for allergies. Adjust the dose for children. As the allergies subside, you can stop taking the tea.

If you know allergy season is coming, you can take this tea preventatively two weeks before your allergies usually start. Increasing your vitamin C intake at the same time by 500mg daily will also help.

1. Boil one quart of water.

2. Add one heaping teaspoon of dried Nettle.

3. Add one heaping teaspoon of dried Goldenrod.

4. Infuse for 15 minutes.

5. Strain into a clean glass vessel.

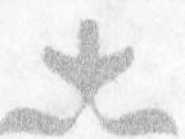

6. Drink three cups, morning, afternoon, and evening.

Most teas store for three to four days.

Tea for Anemia and Fatty Liver (Red Clover Flowers/Yellow Dock Root)

Take this tea for anemia. It also facilitates weight loss. Drink plenty of water while taking this tea.

1. Boil one quart of water.

2. Add one heaping teaspoon of Yellow Dock root.

3. Decoct for 20 minutes (on simmer).

4. Add one heaping teaspoon of Red Clover flowers.

5. Turn off the burner and infuse for 15 minutes.

6. Strain into a clean glass vessel.

Drink three cups, morning, afternoon, and evening

Most teas store for three to four days.

Lemon Balm Tea — Children or Adults
For anxiety, digestion, mild colds

Take this tea for stomach aches, anxiety, mild cold, cough, and sore throat.

1. Boil one quart of water.

2. Add three teaspoons of dried aerial Lemon Balm parts.

3. Infuse for 15 minutes.

4. Strain into a clean glass vessel.

5. Drink three cups, morning, afternoon, and evening. Adjust the dose for children.

Most teas store for three to four days.

Yarrow Tea
for fever, cold, and cough

Yarrow tea will reduce fever, cold, or cough. Yarrow is packed with minerals!

1. Boil one quart of water.

2. Add three teaspoons of dried Yarrow leaves.

3. Infuse for 15 minutes.

4. Strain into a clean glass vessel.

5. Drink three cups, morning, afternoon, and evening. Adjust the dose for children.

Most teas store for three to four days.

Oatstraw Tea
for fatigue and exhaustion

Take this tea for deep restoration after an illness, for short or long-term stress. ***Please note that alongside any other recipe in this book, you can take Oatstraw tea; it will only enhance your remedy and improve your well-being.*** Adjust the dose for children. This formula can be consumed long-term for repair, up to three months.

1. Boil one quart of water.

2. Add three teaspoons of dried Oatstraw.

3. Infuse for 15 minutes

4. Strain into a clean glass vessel

5. Drink three cups, morning, afternoon, and evening

Most teas store for three to four days.

Rose Tea
for depression, relaxation, very mild sore throat, or cold

Take this tea for depression or mild relaxation. Rose tea is also used for very mild colds and sore throats.

1. Boil one quart of water.

2. Add two tablespoons of dried Rose petals.

3. Infuse the petals for 15 minutes.

4. Strain into a clean glass vessel

5. Drink three cups, morning, afternoon, and evening

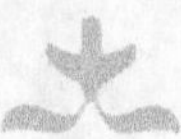

Most teas store for three to four days.

Pine Needles Tea — Children or Adults
for nutrition and immunity

Take this tea to enhance immunity when you are feeling run down. Alternatively, you can take Pine Needles tea with any other herbal protocol for cold cough or flu. It will add extra Vitamins A, B, and C to your diet that absorb quickly.

1. Boil one quart of water.

2. Add ¼ cup chopped Pine Needles.

3. Infuse for 15 minutes.

4. Strain into a clean glass vessel.

5. Drink three cups, morning, afternoon, and evening.

Pine Needles tea is only stored for three days.

12.3 Remedies for Weight Loss and Detoxification

Echinacea Tea
for detoxification, fatigue, and weight loss

Read the Materia Medica section on this herb. Echinacea works by clearing stagnation in the lymphatic system, blood, and liver. When stagnation is cleared it means that detoxification is the result. Detoxification often creates fatigue. It takes energy to move toxins out of the body. ***Please drink extra water when taking this herb.***

1. Boil one quart of water.

2. Add three teaspoons of dried Echinacea leaves and flowers.

3. Infuse the herbs for 15 minutes.

4. Strain into a clean glass vessel

Drink three cups, morning, afternoon, and evening

Most teas store for three to four days.

Daily Nutritive Tea for Weight Loss (Nettle/Rose Hips)

Take this tea for weight loss. It clears stagnation in the liver, nourishes all cells, and has an astringent quality. Astringents, typically sour substances, break down and release fat cells from the body.

1.   Boil one quart of water.

2.   Add one heaping teaspoon of dried Nettle leaves.

3.   Add one heaping teaspoon of dried Rose Hips.

4.   Infuse for 15 minutes.

5.   Strain into a clean glass vessel.

6.   Drink three cups, morning, afternoon, and evening.

Most teas store for three to four days.

12.4 Remedies for Digestive Distress

**Simple Mugwort Tincture
for Worms and Parasites**

Follow the simpling method:

1.   Place four ounces of Mugwort in a clean glass jar.

2.   Cover with the alcohol of your choice, at least 60 proof.

3.   Let the herbs extract for twenty-one days.

4.   Strain the mixture, store it in a glass jar in a cool, dark place.

For an acute situation, take the tincture every three hours for three days to expel the parasites. A tip: you can take hexane-free castor oil capsules to remove parasites and worms in addition to this tincture.

**Anti-Diarrhea Bath for children
(Black Gum Bark or Blackberry
leaves)**

Take this bath instead of a dose of the blackberry tea to help control diarrhoea.

1.   Boil three quarts of water.

   HERBALIST'S GUIDE TO NATIVE AMERICAN REMEDIES

2. Add three heaping tablespoons of dried blackberry leaves.

3. Infuse for 20 minutes.

4. Strain into a clean glass vessel.

5. Run a hot bath.

6. Pour the concentrated tea into a shallow bath.

7. Let the child sit in the tub as usual. The tea will absorb into the skin.

Please note: If you use Black Gum Bark, decoct three heaping tablespoons of the bark in three quarts of water. Strain and add to a shallow child's bath.

12.5 Remedies for Aging and Longevity

Mushroom Broth
for Longevity, Cognition and Stabilizing Mood

Mushroom medicine is a supreme adaptogenic tonic. Mushrooms are full of vitamins, minerals and fiber. They are sustainable and easily grown at home. The most common edible mushrooms contain:

- Beta-glucan-contains fiber, lowers cholesterol and boosts heart health.

- B vitamins-protect nervous system function, metabolize fats, produce red blood cells, stabilize hormones.

- Copper-supports oxygen delivery throughout the body, bone and nerve maintenance.

- Niacin-revives the skin and restores digestive function.

- Potassium-sustains heart, muscle, and nerve function.

- Selenium-metabolizes damaged cells and boosts immunity.

A broth functions in the same way as tea.

1. Chop three edible mushrooms of your choice.

2. Boil them in a cup of water for fifteen minutes.

3. Add whatever spice you like.

Strain the mixture and save the mushrooms for cooking. You can drink one to three cups of mushroom broth daily.

Alternatively, you can saute mushrooms and add two tablespoons to your daily vegetables. Most grocery stores carry medicinal mushrooms like shiitake, or maitake. Mushrooms have very similar properties and nutritional value. You can even use crimini mushrooms, portobello or white button mushrooms regularly in your diet. While you learn about foraging mushrooms, at least experiment with edible mushrooms in your kitchen.

Oak Bark Tea
for kidney infections and kidney stones

1. Boil one quart of water.

2. Add one tablespoon of Oak Bark.

3. Decoct for 20 minutes.

4. Strain into a clean glass vessel.

5. Drink three cups daily.

Most teas store for three to four days.

Oak Bark Compress
for burns and cuts

1. Make the Oak Bark decoction recipe above.

2. Rather than drinking it, you will soak a 12" by 12" cloth in the tea after the tea has cooled slightly.

3. Wring the cloth out, fold it into thirds, and place it on the painful or inflamed area for 20 minutes.

4. Repeat throughout the day as often as needed.

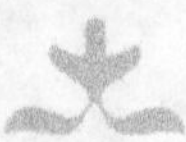

Acorn Pudding
for Rehabilitation and Restoration

1. Gather 4 cups of acorns and shell them.

2. Soak the meat of the acorn in water overnight. The soaking process will release most of the tannins.

3. Put the acorn meat through a strainer the following day and rinse it thoroughly. Puree this with a bit of water in the blender. Put the puree in a small pot and simmer for 20 minutes. Add honey and ghee or butter to your taste.

Take three small servings of this or more daily, or as needed for restoration and nourishment. This pudding and Oatstraw Tea combine well as restorative remedies that build strength and nutrition.

Cattail Poultice
for burns, bruises, and inflammation

(You can use this poultice in addition to Arnica oil and the Devil's Club tea following an injury or surgery.)

1. Collect one cup of root.

2. Boil it for 15 minutes and then drain the water.

3. Mash the root and make a paste.

4. Let it cool to touch and spread the paste on a square cloth 12" by 12" in the middle.

5. Fold the edges into the middle and place the flat side on the affected area for 20 minutes.

Repeat throughout the day in an acute case or two times daily for chronic pain, bruising, or inflammation.

California Poppy Remedy
for adult anxiety

1. Gather one cup of flowers and seeds.

2. Place in a clean glass jar.

3. Cover with alcohol.

4. Let the mixture sit for twenty-one days.

5. Strain the mixture into a clean glass jar or two-ounce dropper bottles.

6. Store in a cool dark place.

Take 1 "or one dropper full two to three times daily for anxiety or insomnia.

Blackberry Soup
for reducing fatigue, gaining strength, and blood sugar stabilization

1. Place one and ½ cups of blackberries in a small pot.

2. Add ⅓ teaspoon cinnamon.

3. Simmer for ten minutes and mash the berries with a potato masher.

Cool and consume, just like a soup. If you have the soup in the evening, it will help stabilize blood sugar levels throughout the night and reduce cravings the following day. One bowl of the soup long-term will help support adrenal function.

Sage Oral Swish
for a Toothache or Teeth Whitening

1. Make a cup of Sage tea using the standard dosage method of 1 teaspoon of dried herb to one cup of boiling water.

2. Let the tea steep for 15 minutes.

3. Strain the tea.

4. Swish one tablespoon of the tea in your mouth for 15 minutes. You can also hold the tea with your mouth over the affected tooth for several seconds. Then continue to swish.

5. Spit the tea out.

6. Save the remainder of the tea in a glass jar in the refrigerator.

7. Repeat the process until you feel the pain subside.

Dental pain may be a sign that further care is required. Please see the following for a more comprehensive perspective on holistic dental care.[7]

12.6 Remedies for Beauty

Perform the following routine in the evening.

Rose/Sage Face Steam

Place one teaspoon each of Rose petals and Sage in a small pot of hot steaming water. Make a tent over your head with a hand towel and put your face one foot above the pot. Allow the vapors to open your pores for a few minutes.

After steaming, dry the skin and apply the Nettle face pack below.

Nettle Face Mask (Green face mask to detoxify and regenerate)

1. Put one teaspoon of Nettle powder in a small bowl.

2. Add four teaspoons of French Green Clay.

3. Add three drops of lavender essential oil.

4. Mix the ingredients into a paste.

Take one teaspoon of the paste and spread it over your face without coming too close to the eyes. Let it dry until it begins to crack. Take a hot steaming washcloth, ring it out and remove your mask. Repeat until you remove the mask. Proceed with your usual routine.

Overnight, apply some of the **Rose massage oil** as a deep emollient.

---

7   Alexander, Leslie M., PhD, RH (AHG) and Linda A. Straub-Bruce, BS Ed, RDH, Vermont: Healing Arts Press, 2014.

12.7 Remedies for Sexual and Reproductive Health

Please review the Ginseng tea and Rosemary Hair oil recipes listed above. You may want to add both to your routine.

Please note for the following recipe, if dried blackberries are not available, you could substitute blueberries, raspberries, or goji berries.

Menstrual Formula for Teens and Adults
Black Cohosh/ Saw Palmetto/Oatstraw/ Dried Blackberry Tincture

1. Place equal parts, ¼ cup each of Black Cohosh/ Saw Palmetto/ Oatstraw, and dried Blackberries in a quart jar.

2. Use the simpling method and cover with the alcohol of your choice.

3. Let the tincture extract for twenty-one days. Strain it and pour it into a glass jar or two-ounce dropper bottles.

4. Take 1" or one dropper full three times daily, morning, afternoon, and evening.

Sexual Tonic for Women
Rose/Lemon Balm/ Chamomile/Mint

This recipe is a tonic nervine and mood-enhancing tea. It works well when combined with the Rose massage oil. Remember that sexual desire is often enhanced by stress reduction, balancing lifestyle issues, and increasing self-esteem.

1. Boil two quarts of water.

2. Add 1/2 tablespoon each dried Rose, Lemon Balm, and Chamomile.

3. Add one teaspoon of Mint

4. Infuse for 15 minutes

5. Strain into a clean glass vessel

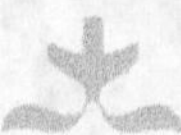

6. Drink three cups, morning, afternoon, and evening

Most teas store for three to four days.

Take a break periodically from this tonic for four days and then resume for long-term use.

Sexual Tonics for Men

**Ginseng/Hops/Oatstraw/ Dried Blackberry Tincture
for erectile dysfunction, strength, endurance**

1. Place equal parts, ¼ cup each of Ginseng/Hops/Oatstraw, and dried Blackberries in a quart jar.

2. Use the simpling method and cover with the alcohol of your choice.

Let the tincture extract for twenty-one days. Strain it and pour it into a glass jar or 2-ounce dropper bottle.
Take 1" or one dropper full three times daily, morning, afternoon, and evening.

**Saw Palmetto/Hops Tonic
for fatigue, lethargy, anxiety, endurance**

1. Follow the same formula and dosage in the recipe above.

2. Substitute Saw Palmetto for Ginseng during the preparation.

**Rose Massage Oil
for relaxation and romance**

1. In a quart-sized jar, place 1 cup Rose petals.

2. Cover the petals entirely with whatever oil you choose (olive, almond, avocado, apricot are good choices)

3. Cover the jar with a lid.

4. Store in a cool, dark place for thirty to forty days. It takes a long time for oil extractions to complete.

5. Shake the jar a couple of times a week to mix your ingredients.

6. After the extraction is finished, strain the oil into a strainer lined with cheesecloth that sits over a bowl.

7. After the oil drips through the cloth, gather the edges of the cloth. Twist and squeeze all of the oil out into the bowl.

8. Pour the finished extraction into a glass jar.

9. Store in a cool, dark place. Oleolites have a fair degree of shelf stability and will last for a couple of years when stored properly.

**Horsetail/Uva Ursi Tea
for Urinary tract infections**

Take this tea for urinary tract infections. The horsetail is soothing, while Uva Ursi is highly astringent. It also helps to alternate this tea with ¼ cup of unsweetened cranberry juice throughout the day. Take this tea for three days. See a practitioner if your symptoms do not improve.

1. Boil one quart of water.

2. Add one heaping teaspoon of dried aerial Horsetail parts

3. Add one heaping teaspoon of dried Uva Ursi

4. Infuse for 15 minutes

5. Strain into a clean glass vessel

6. Drink three cups, morning, afternoon, and evening

Most teas store for three to four days.

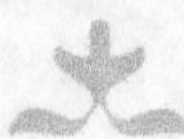

13   Conclusion

Great! I'm so glad that you had the chance to read the whole book! The moment has come to take action and start preparing your remedies if you have not done so already. Are there any ideas lingering in the back of your mind about practices you would like to pursue? Curiosity and interest are valuable prerequisites for any type of success in life! So far, we have provided you with the knowledge and the tools to either start or deepen your practice in herbal medical pursuits.

Deciding to familiarize yourself with Native American practices involves studying their herbal remedy preparation techniques alongside their cultural traditions. At this point, just by reading this book, you have affirmed the importance of the mind-body connection. It is critical for health. Seeing how our lives and surroundings benefit from different perspectives is invaluable. A new perspective yields a pause for reflection, perhaps embracing a new worldview or even a totally different focus in life. The power to choose our reality and shape the world in which we live rests within us.

We emphasize that all aspects of self-care are essential for a balanced life. Now you understand 40 herbs and plants Native Americans use to enhance and heal. The base provided is comprehensive enough to cover most basic (family) ailments. However, we must stress again, and again that if an ailment continues or worsens, or you react to an herb, do not hesitate to contact a professional herbalist, qualified holistic practitioner, or doctor for a second opinion.

Now it is your turn! Start small and continue forever towards a healthy and balanced self.

We wish you all the best.

Loved the book?

A quick review on 'Goodreads' helps small authors & booksellers grow!

- SCAN ME -

https://www.goodreads.com/review/edit/62107173

STRESS RESILIENCE WORKBOOK WITH SEASONAL HEALING HERBAL INFUSIONS

16 Tools for Balanced Health & Focused Energy through Nutrition Matching your Body Type & Mindfulness Practice

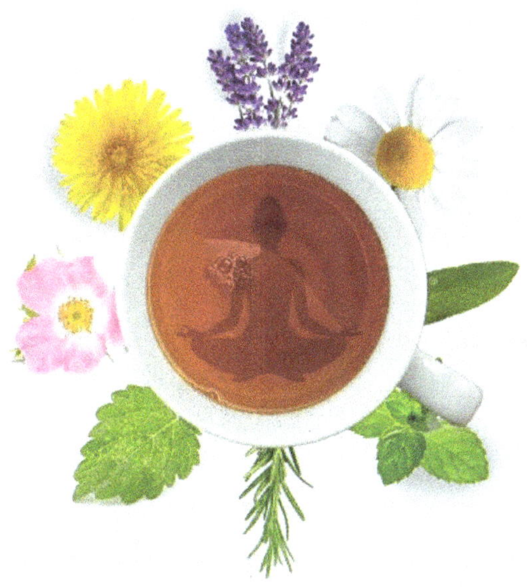

Breathe a stress-free life. This book is full of actionable advice to help you balance your seasonal body reactions, break the stress cycle, and achieve true positivity. - The keys lie within yourself – understanding your body's natural rhythms and learning to work with them.

https://www.leafinprint.com/books

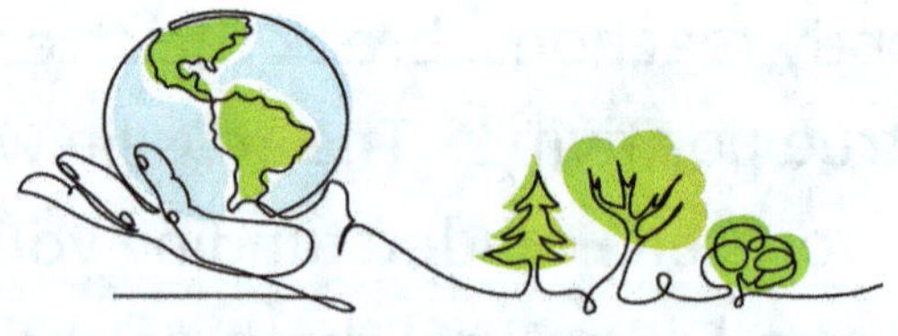

Version v4 - 9.2025